OXFORD MEDICAL PUBLICATIONS

Addiction: Processes of Change

Addiction: Processes of Change

SOCIETY FOR THE STUDY OF ADDICTION MONOGRAPH NO. 3

Edited by

GRIFFITH EDWARDS

Honorary Director
Addiction Research Unit
National Addiction Centre
London

and

MALCOLM LADER

Head of Psychopharmacology Section
Department of Psychiatry
Institute of Psychiatry
University of London

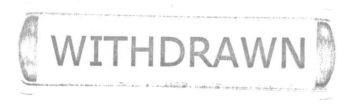

Oxford   New York   Tokyo
OXFORD UNIVERSITY PRESS
1994

Oxford University Press, Walton Street, Oxford OX2 6DP

Oxford   New York

Athens   Auckland   Bangkok   Bombay
Calcutta   Cape Town   Dar es Salaam   Delhi
Florence   Hong Kong   Istanbul   Karachi
Kuala Lumpur   Madras   Madrid   Melbourne
Mexico City   Nairobi   Paris   Singapore
Taipei   Tokyo   Toronto
and associated companies in
Berlin   Ibadan

Oxford is a trade mark of Oxford University Press

Published in the United States
by Oxford University Press Inc., New York

A catalogue record for this book is available from the British Library

Library of Congress Cataloging in Publication Data
Addiction : processes of change / edited by Griffith Edwards and
Malcolm H. Lader. — 1st ed.
p.   cm. — (Oxford medical publications)   (Society for the
Study of Addiction monograph; no. 3)
Proceedings of a meeting held in April 1992 at Cumberland Lodge in
Windsor Great Park, Berkshire, UK.
Includes bibliographical references and index.
1. Substance abuse—Congresses.   I. Edwards. Griffith.
II. Lader, Malcolm Harold.   III. Series.   IV. Series: Monograph
(Society for the Study of Addiction); no. 3.
[DNLM: 1. Substance Dependence—psychology—congresses.
2. Substance Dependence—therapy—congresses.   W1 M05558L no. 3
1994 / WM 270 A22392 1994]
RC563.2.A29   1994   616.86—dc20   94—11037

ISBN 0 19 262433 4

Typeset by Apex Products, Singapore
Printed in Great Britain on acid-free paper by
Biddles Ltd. Guildford & King's Lynn

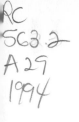
Preface

The Society for the Study of Addiction was originally founded in 1884 as the Society for the Study and Cure of Inebriety. It held annual meetings and, from the start, published a journal which, after several changes of title, now appears monthly as *Addiction*. It is now regarded as the leading journal in the topic.

The Society has broadened its interests to include all substances of abuse. It has also broadened its membership over the years to represent a wide range of professions, expertise, and background. It now has a membership of over 500. Its annual meetings are very successful, each focusing on a particular theme, but also including communications from the membership.

To complement these open meetings, a small meeting is held every two years at Cumberland Lodge, in Windsor Great Park, Berkshire, UK, in a setting of great historical interest and in beautiful countryside. These meetings are limited to invited participants, world experts in their areas of research, who debate informally a topic selected for its broad appeal to those working across a range of problems. The first subject chosen was 'The nature of drug dependence': the meeting was held in April 1988, and the proceedings published as the first in this series of monographs by Oxford University Press in 1990. The second meeting took as its theme 'Substance misuse—what makes problems?'; the proceedings of this meeting held in April 1990 were published in 1992.

The third meeting was devoted to the topic of 'Addiction—multiple processes of change'. A carefully chosen group of participants from a wide range of disciplines and research interests met at Cumberland Lodge in April 1992. Papers were pre-circulated and briefly introduced, and as much time as possible was reserved for full and frank discussions which developed those topics.

The participants then submitted revised manuscripts which form the bulk of this monograph. A few additional topics were identified and papers commissioned to augment the original chapters.

We are grateful to all participants for giving up time preparing these excellent contributions and attending the meeting. Our thanks are due to Mrs Lily Hughes, the Administrative Officer of the Society, for her excellent organization of the meeting, and to Mrs Pat Davies for her expert editorial assistance. Finally, we are grateful to Oxford University Press for once again publishing the Society's Monograph.

London   G. E.
November 1993   M. L.

Contents

PART IV. PROCESSES OF CHANGE: MAKING THE CONNECTION BETWEEN THEORY AND CLINICAL PRACTICE

Contributors

ROBIN DAVIDSON, *Area Clinical Psychologist, Northern Health and Social Services, Holywell Hospital, Antrim, Northern Ireland, UK.*

MARY ALISON DURAND, *Research Psychologist, Addiction Research Unit, National Addiction Centre, London, UK.*

GRIFFITH EDWARDS, *Honorary Director, Addiction Research Unit, National Addiction Centre, London, UK.*

ROBERTA FERRENCE, *Senior Scientist, Social Evaluation and Research, Addiction Research Foundation, Toronto, Canada.*

CHRISTINE GODFREY, *Senior Research Fellow, Centre for Health Economics, University of York, UK.*

MARTIN JARVIS, *ICRF Health Behaviour Unit, Addiction Sciences Building, London, UK.*

HARALD K.-H. KLINGEMANN, *Research Director, Swiss Institute for the Prevention of Alcohol and Drug Problems, Lausanne, Switzerland.*

MALCOLM LADER, *Head, Psychopharmacology Section, Department of Psychiatry, Institute of Psychiatry, London, UK.*

DAVID NUTT, *Senior Research Fellow in Mental Health and Pharmacology, Psychopharmacology Unit, University of Bristol, UK.*

CHARLES R. SCHUSTER, *Senior Research Scientist, Addiction Research Center, National Institute on Drug Abuse, Rockville, Maryland, USA.*

REGINALD G. SMART, *Head, Social Epidemiology, Addiction Research Foundation, Toronto, Canada.*

JOHN STRANG, *Getty Senior Lecturer in the Addictions and Deputy Director, Addiction Research Unit, National Addiction Centre, London, UK.*

STEPHEN SUTTON, *Senior Scientist and Senior Lecturer in Social Psychology, ICRF Health Behaviour Unit, Addiction Sciences Building, London, UK.*

COLIN TAYLOR, *Statistician, National Addiction Centre, and Senior Lecturer in Departments of Psychiatry and Biostatistics, Institute of Psychiatry, London, UK.*

Part I.

Introduction

1

Change as a dominant theme in science

MALCOLM LADER

INTRODUCTION

In this introductory paper, the scene will be set for the other contributors to support, refute, or elaborate on some aspects of this important topic. Various aspects of change will be touched on, by necessity only superficially; many will be taken up in other chapters in greater depth and wider erudition. My approach is the credo of a jobbing scientist: we should seize every opportunity to study spontaneous change (Nature's experiment); we should develop dependable methods of inducing change in the systems which interest us; we must investigate the mechanisms which subserve change; and finally we must attempt to ascribe cause to the effects which we have studied.

Science is a body of knowledge whose prime purpose is to allow us to predict the course of future events. In more precise terms, it allows us to anticipate change by means of predictive equations. However, the way in which scientists do this is debatable. The success of the predictions is undisputed in practical terms. The condition of man on planet Earth has changed out of recognition in the past few millennia, particularly in the past few centuries and amazingly so in the past few decades. Two major advances stand out: the harnessing of unimaginable amounts of energy to facilitate, amplify, and extend human endeavours, and the ability, by means of molecular biology, to influence our own destinies. But how do we arrive at these highly successful predictive algorithms?

The traditional way in which scientific knowledge develops is identified with Francis Bacon (1605). He realized that an unstructured set of observations was unhelpful. He suggested that the observations had first to be categorized and then used as the basis of an inductive hypothesis. From this hypothesis one should be able to deduce logically future events and then by observing those events, see whether the hypothesis is supported or refuted. If refuted, then another hypothesis must be constructed. However, an hypothesis can never be proved, only fail to be disproved. In other words, all hypotheses are provisional statements of the natural laws of the universe.

Modern philosophers have challenged this view of the logical development of scientific hypotheses and predictions. Karl Popper (1968), the most distinguished member of this school, argued strongly that the building of hypotheses is part intuition and part rational, and only the testing of an hypothesis follows totally rational principles. Taken to its extreme, hypothesis construction is a branch of aesthetics!

However, the role of the fortuitous observation is generally underplayed. A change can be observed as an isolated instance. However, if a reproducible event accompanies that change, then the fortuitous observation of that association may set in train a series of firstly spontaneous observations and later controlled interventions involving careful manipulation of that event or events. The later observations will, of course, no longer be fortuitous but will be directed by scientific questions, that is by hypotheses of various types. One observer might favour one hypothesis because of his previous experience and training. Further observations of change will be highly selective, depending on the hypothesis generated.

Scientific observations depend on the order of events, that is unidirectional time is an important assumption. Biologists and chemists work to this assumption. Physicists, particularly cosmologists, have much more cavalier views of a phenomenon we take for granted. Some cosmological theories do not assume time to be unidirectional and dependable. Leaving aside these reservations, in biology we believe from our observations of change that 'like objects placed in like circumstances will always produce like effects' (Hume 1748). But even this has been questioned by the author of that quote, David Hume. Hume (1748) acknowledged that:

For all inferences from experience suppose, as their foundation, that the future will resemble the past and similar powers will be conjoined with similar sensible qualities. If there be any suspicion that the course of nature may change and the past be no rule for the future, all experience becomes useless and can give rise to no inference or conclusion. It is impossible, therefore, that any argument from experience can prove this resemblance of the past to the future, since all arguments are founded on the supposition of that resemblance.

However, this defeatist although highly logical argument is founded on the premise in the first part of the second sentence that one can suppose that the laws of nature can change. This is a belief like any other: if one has religious beliefs, more specifically that miracles can happen, then predictions about the future outside that belief system are impossible. If one accepts the inviolability of natural laws, then predictions are possible but theology is not. If one attempts a compromise, that predictions are almost always possible but occasional miracles do occur, then one has to specify under what circumstances miracles can be predicted.

EPIDEMIOLOGICAL APPROACH

This is a very large and technical subject and I shall confine myself to one very important example, smoking and carcinoma of the bronchus. The initial observations linking the two were of an increase in the incidence of carcinoma of the bronchus which paralleled, with a time lag, the increase in cigarette smoking in the general population. However, many other variables had also increased, for example, the number of motor vehicles on the roads. Apologists for the tobacco industry put up all sorts of alternative explanations of varying degrees of face validity. Thus observations of change had led to an hypothesis and although most medical and scientific people believed the hypothesis to be sound, practical action was slow and halting.

Important, perhaps crucial evidence, of the link came from observations of the smoking habits of doctors. The usage of cigarettes among medical practitioners fell substantially and was followed after a time lag by a marked reduction in the incidence of lung cancer. Few, if any, of the alternative hypotheses could be entertained—the link between smoking and cancer was firmly established even if the causative chain was not properly worked out. The statistical probability that the link was a fortuitous one was vanishingly small. Only the tobacco industry apologists denied the unassailable strength of the hypothesis. In this instance, changes against the general trend provided extremely persuasive evidence.

BIOMEDICAL APPROACH

The third aspect I shall outline concerns the formal study of changes induced by therapeutic interventions. The evaluation of change induced by treatment accounts for much of the decision making of everyday clinical practice. It combines naturalistic observation of the individual patient with past personal experience and clinical acumen. However, many biases can creep into the assessment of change and clinical scientists have expended much effort and ingenuity into devising ways of assessing change as objectively as possible. In the dependence field, the treatment process is usually complex and intricate with a plethora of biological and social forces acting on the patient quite independently of overt factors such as the administration of a pill. Nevertheless, the change can be measured; it is the confident ascribing of the change to antecedent factors which is difficult. Variables such as the expectations of the patient, his reaction to contact with the clinic, the nature of the interaction between patient and doctor, and the expertise and attitudes of the doctor are all instrumental in modifying change induced by the specific treatment of interest. Some of these issues will now be addressed.

Multiple change

No treatment results in an isolated change. One change in particular— the 'wanted effect'—may be the focus of interest, but many other changes will occur. Some will be welcome, so called wanted effects, others will be unwanted. Many side effects may be apparent to the patient and cause discomfort, some may be serious and endanger health. Others may be subtle and apparent only on special testing, for example, cognitive effects of some drugs of dependence. All these individual effects may have different dose thresholds, different latencies before developing, and differ from individual to individual.

Dose effects

The change effected by a treatment is usually proportional to the intensity and frequency of that treatment, that is its dosage parameters. However, typically a lower threshold dose exists below which no change can be detected, and an upper ceiling dose beyond which no further change occurs. Between these limits an orderly progression of change should follow each increment in the treatment. If this does not occur then some other important factors are intervening and are being overlooked.

Initial level effects

One major and eventually unresolved problem in the measurement of change is the effect of the initial level. Put simply, is a change from 1 to 2 the same in biological, or even physicochemical terms, as a change from 11 to 12? Assuming a linear scale, in absolute terms the changes are the same, but in relative terms, one is a doubling, the other a change of less than a tenth of the initial value. There are many examples in biology of responses being dependent on the initial value (Wilder 1958). Experimental studies of emotional reactions in humans provide numerous instances. For example, Gardos *et al.* (1968) rated student volunteers according to their habitual anxiety measured by a self-rating question-naire. Their responses to placebo and to the benzodiazepines, oxazepam and chlordiazepoxide, were then studied. Subjects who were very anxious experienced a considerable reduction in anxiety following the drugs, those who were moderately anxious had a smaller reduction, and those who were calm actually became anxious after receiving benzodiazepines. Interestingly, those whose anxiety was greatly relieved by chlordiazep-oxide experienced increased anger and aggressiveness. Obviously, in clinical practice, one would not knowingly give an anxiolytic to someone who was not anxious, but histrionic display might be mistaken for anxiety and benzodiazepines might also be given for another purpose, for example to ease muscle spasm. Aggressiveness was an early reported behavioural 'side effect' of the benzodiazepines and has been demonstrated, along with other 'paradoxical' effects, in many experimental studies.

Individual variation

Individual variation is an acknowledgement, however covert, of our ignorance concerning the factors governing change. When a change is larger or smaller than that predicted, we ascribe it to individual varia-tion, a totally circular argument. We have to examine this variability and attempt to minimize it by evaluating such factors as age, sex, body habitus, nutrition, degree of physical activity, and a host of psychological factors such as motivation and expectations. Many of these issues will be addressed by later speakers.

Milieu effects

Change is also profoundly influenced by the setting in which it occurs or is induced. It is a common social observation that the effects of alcohol can be very different when it is taken in quiet solitude than when taken in a social group and the effects are conditioned by what is going on in the group. A 'sedative' agent can readily become a 'stimulant' leading to overactivity, gregariousness, and social disinhibition. Some benzodiazepines, particularly chlordiazepoxide, lower the threshold for hostile feelings which may only become manifest in social interactions (Salzman *et al.* 1974). Environmental influences have been detected in schizophrenic patients treated at home where the emotional atmosphere has an important effect on the relapse rate and the effectiveness of antipsychotics. In families with high 'expressed emotion' relapse is more frequent and the protective effect of maintenance antipsychotics can be demonstrated. In more equable families relapse is much less common and the ability of these drugs to prevent it (compared with placebo) is not apparent (Vaughn and Leff 1976).

Placebo effects

Milieu and other influences can modify the actions of drugs which have known effects. It is, therefore, not too surprising that inert substances, 'dummies' or 'placebos', can produce changes. Indeed, placebos have many of the 'pharmacological' properties already described (Wolf 1959; Shapiro and Morris 1978; Joyce 1962) including dose effects, time effects, unwanted effects, they may cause dependence and their use may be accompanied by relevant bodily changes: for example endorphin release probably mediates placebo-induced analgesia (Levine *et al*. 1978). Placebo effects are determined by many interacting factors in the treatment situation and it is not possible to state what factors on their own will be consistently associated with response to placebo. There is, for example, no evidence that placebo reactors have a particular type of personality or that they will consistently react. Placebo reactions may occur even though the individual knows that he is receiving an inert substance and accepts that to be the case and, perhaps against common-sense expectation, relief from physical and emotional discomfort is more likely with a placebo at intense pain levels than mild ones. The hopes, fears, and expectations of the individual patient are critical and in most societies much is expected of pills and potions.

Therapist effects

Finally, the influence of the person attempting to effect change is very important. The social interaction at the focus of treatment is, of course, the doctor—patient relationship and it would not be surprising if this affected the response to drug treatment. Obviously, many factors could be involved, such as the doctor's enthusiasm for the treatment, his capacity to encourage and support the patient, the degree of psycho-therapeutic involvement, and so on. Clinical trials in which these have been measured, albeit rather crudely, have shown some influence on the activity of anxiolytic, antidepressant, and antipsychotic drugs (Joyce 1962; Rickels *et al*. 1971; Shader *et al*. 1971). Inevitably perhaps, in view of the subtle changes in treatment settings, the effect of the therapist is not easily replicated even by the same investigators. Enthusiastic therapists may be found to augment drug effects in one study and to reduce them in another. This 'will-o'-the wisp' character makes it difficult to harness such forces, but it is unwise not to recognize their presence.

CONCLUSIONS

Change, either spontaneously observed or induced under carefully controlled conditions, is the bedrock phenomenon upon which much scientific theory and practice is based. In biology a variety of factors may hamper interpretation of that change into cause-and-effect terms. Simple evaluation in terms of association is a useful first step but may be misleading. The transition of a topic from natural history observations to active intervention studies is a sign of the growing maturity of that topic. Addiction is an area where a great number of biosocial factors interact. Nevertheless, the undoubted complexity should not deter us from attempting carefully controlled studies in which one variable is altered at a time. Of course, several dependent measures may need monitoring but the powerful nature of the resultant data, both in terms of theoretical insights and practical advances, usually repays us all our efforts.

REFERENCES

Bacon, F. (1605). *The advancement of learning*, Book 2, Section VIII.

Gardos, G., Dimascio, A., Saltzman, C., and Shader, R. I. (1968). Differential actions of chlordiazepoxide and oxazepam on hostility. *Archives of General Psychiatry*, **18**, 757–60.

Hume, D. (1748). *An inquiry concerning human understanding*, Section 4, Part 2, p. 51. Bobbs-Merrill, New York, 1955.

Joyce, C. R. B. (1962). Differences between physicians as revealed by clinical trials. *Proceedings of the Royal Society of Medicine*, **55**, 776–8.

Levine, J. D., Gordon, N. C., and Fields, H. L. (1978). The mechanisms of placebo analgesia. *Lancet*, **ii**, 654–7.

Popper, K. (1968). *The logic of scientific discovery*. Hutchinson, London.

Rickels, K., Lipman, R. S., Park, L. C., Covi, L., Uhlenhuth, E. H., and Mock, J. E. (1971). Drug, doctor warmth and clinic setting in the symptomatic response to minor tranquillisers. *Psychopharmacologia*, **20**, 128–52.

Salzman, C., Kochansky, G. E., Shader, R. I., Porrino, L. J., Harmatz, J. S., and Swett, C. P. (1974). Chlordiazepoxide-induced hostility in a small group setting. *Archives of General Psychiatry*, **31**, 401–5.

Shader, R. I., Grinspoon, L., Harmatz, J. S., and Ewart, J. R. (1971). The therapist variable. *American Journal of Psychiatry*, **127**, 49–52.

Shapiro, A. K. and Morris, L. A. (1978). The placebo effect in medical and psychological therapies. In *Handbook of psychotherapy and behavior change*, (2nd edn) (ed. S. L. Garfield and A. E. Bergin), pp. 208–19. John Wiley, New York.

Vaughn, C. and Leff, J. P. (1976). The influence of family and social factors on the course of psychiatric illness: a comparison of schizophrenic and depressed neurotic patients. *British Journal of Psychiatry*, **124**, 784–96.

Wilder, J. (1958). Modern psychophysiology and the law of initial value. *American Journal of Psychotherapy*, **12**, 199–221.

Wolf, S. (1959). The pharmacology of placebos. *Pharmacology Review*, **11**, 689–704.

Part II.

Science and understanding of change at the personal level

2

Alcohol, drug, and tobacco dependence: charting and comparing the likelihood and time-course of relapse and recovery

COLIN TAYLOR

INTRODUCTION

The contents of this chapter focus on the central point of the title, the expression 'time-course', and without any attempt to cover the field systematically or review the literature it makes some highly selective and idiosyncratic points about change and process. As examples it uses data from some longer term addiction studies, often ones with some personal connection, with the aim of conveying a general sense of a perspective on change and process. As it proceeds, the focus moves from the minutiae of transitions from abstinence to drug consumption and to abstinence again, moving to one which uses the other end of the telescope in order to give a view of the overall lifespan of drug users and the processes we might need to postulate.

To begin, the basic characterization of the processes of abstaining and relapsing is to imagine that these phenomena are conceived as a sequence:

cessation–abstinence–relapse–consumption–secondary cessation...

with an option to repeat the cycle *ad mortem*. The cessation is usually associated with a treatment episode, although of course there is no requirement for this to be the case and it may follow a cessation attempt which we would usually and probably erroneously term spontaneous. The cessation is regarded as a particular point in time as is the point of relapse, usually considered strictly identifiable as the last and first administration of the drug. Recognition of a continuing process of cessation and relapse underlying these visible discontinuities allows some leeway in the precise definition of these points.

Within this schema, outcome of the treatment episode or the spontaneous cessation attempt is taken as the state which obtains at an arbitrary agreed time-point; in the absence of the rather forlorn hope that there will not be much change after the chosen outcome point, outcome is usually taken as a set of results indexed by time: 6-month outcome, 12-month outcome, and so forth.

In order to facilitate discussion it is necessary to draw an immediate distinction between models for the substantive phenomena involved, which are logical structures usually specifying causal connections, and mathematical or statistical models, which are concerned with formulating these in a way which can be matched against recorded facts. The former, substantive models—one might call them phenomenal models—can be regarded as dealing with the logical connections between concepts such as addiction memory, behavioural conditioning, and decision making, as well as incorporating social, genetic, personality, and motivational influences. Much has been written about these models but this chapter concentrates upon the way they resolve into mathematical models in the time domain.

CESSATION AND RELAPSE

Characterizing the risk of relapse

There are probably no mathematical models—and none of which the author is aware—that seek to predict outcome in the sense of deterministic prediction, with a failure so to do attributed to mis-specification, or incomplete specification, of the model. Statistical analyses in the past have sought a purely statistical prediction of outcome status at a fixed point in time. This would be achieved for example by a simple regression model—or with slightly more sophistication, a logistic regression model—relating the outcome to a clutch of predictors. These analyses would seem to shed little light on the process of change: replacing the outcome status 'abstinence' by a refinement using the criterion of 'sustained abstinence since treatment' equally sheds little light on the concept of process. It could be argued that generally the smoking field has been the last to let go of this type of approach, and so it is fitting that it also seems to be the field in which the more process-orientated analyses are now being used.

The current fashion is to put these analyses within the framework of survival models ('survival' in the statistical jargon, or 'sustained

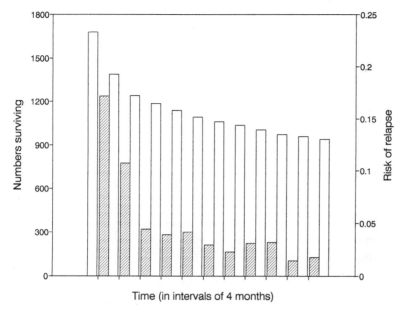

FIG. 2.1   MRFIT data: survival and risk function (after Fan and Elketroussi 1989).

abstinence' in the current context) which fundamentally requires the recording of the length of time until change of status. This has the effect of shifting the focus from 'status at a predetermined point' to 'length of time until change'. Thus a typical example is this set of data from the Multiple Risk Factor Intervention Trial (MRFIT) programme in the USA (Fig. 2.1, after Fan and Elketroussi 1989). The horizontal axis in the figure charts the passage of time; the vertical left-hand scale counts the number of survivors at the end of each time period (each are 4 months in length), represented by the lighter columns in the figure. The columns thus depict a standard survival curve: the numbers surviving without relapse to each subsequent time point.

The results giving numbers surviving at successive points in time, are shown here supplemented with the risk curve, also referred to as the hazard curve, which gives the probability of relapsing at any point after treatment, *given that* abstinence had been sustained up to that point. Thus the darker columns, measured against the right-hand scale in the diagram, show for each period the number of relapsers in that period as a proportion of the current survivors at that time. This risk function constitutes the main information on the time-course of the *process* of

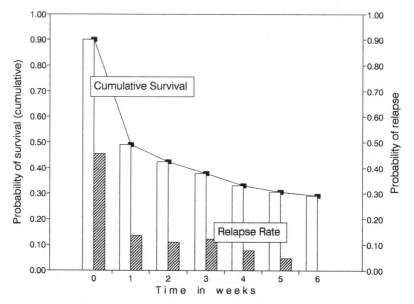

FIG. 2.2 Opiate relapse (adapted from Bradley 1989; Gossop *et al.* 1989). Lighter columns show the proportion of survivors at each point, darker columns show the proportion relapsing each week. For further details see text.

relapse, in that it gives risk information about exactly those people exposed to the risk of relapse, and gives it as it changes at each point in time. Incidentally, it is worth noting that the proportion, shown in this figure, still surviving in abstinence after four years is artificially high and is a consequence of the the way the subjects in this data set have been selected. Survival rates will of course vary with programme and clientele, but one would expect generally to find one-year sustained abstinence to vary between say 15 and 35 per cent. The relevant point about the observed time-course of events as depicted in this study is that the *probability of relapsing* decreases overall in the survivor group as time progresses. It might *be debated* whether or not the second half of the figure shows a decreasing or a flattened risk, but the overall picture is clear: as time progresses, relapse in the group is less likely.

This observation is relatively common and is demonstrated further in a study of opiate relapse (Fig. 2.2 Bradley 1989; Gossop *et al.* 1989). In this figure the risk curve has been superimposed on the diagram of the survival curve as originally published and from which it was calculated, so the figures are somewhat approximate. The left-hand scale shows the proportion of survivors at each point (lighter columns) forming

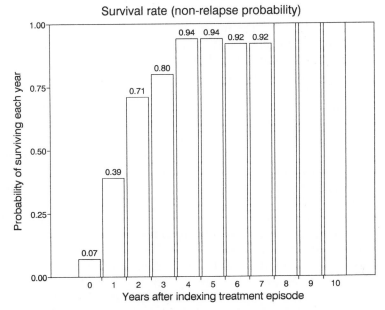

FIG. 2.3 Survival rates (from Taylor *et al*. 1985) after alcohol intake.

the survival curve and also the proportion relapsing each week (darker columns) forming the risk curve. The risks of relapse here are noticeably higher (about 10 per cent per week) than in the smoking relapse study (less than 5 per cent per 4-month period), again possibly due to the selection criteria in the latter data set, but the same downward trend in risk of relapse is apparent. It is important to note that the risk curve, unlike a survival curve, is free to rise or take on any other pattern with the passage of time but in fact it falls. Note that the time scale is very different in this study, its shortness reflecting perhaps both the nature of the treatment clientele as well as the difference between nicotine and opiates.

Again, in a previously published paper on alcohol relapse (Fig. 2.3, Taylor *et al*. 1985) a similar pattern shows, although here the time scale is in years rather than in weeks. In this figure the probability of surviving rather than the probability of relapsing is depicted, but an imagined inverting of the vertical axis reveals a declining probability of relapse which parallels the risk curves for drug and nicotine relapse.

It is clear that in these analyses a strictly deterministic model of the process of relapse is not attempted, but rather the statistical model is formulated as an explicitly stochastic model: that is, one which specifies a probability of relapse at any point after cessation, and deliberately ascribes to unspecified chance whether or not an actual relapse is realized for any given individual. The image created by the model is of a person pushed out of treatment with a predisposition or vulnerability to re- lapse characterized by this risk function—a predisposition which may change over the immediate future—and who is subject to the random buffetings of fortune that will determine his or her fate.

It is worth emphasizing at this juncture the nature of the data these figures display. They are calculated from information on the timing of a *first relapse*, however defined, and show on average how the risk for *the group* changes over time. There is a need to be wary in exactly how this is interpreted for each individual. The model of an individual having a predisposition to relapse which diminishes over time is appeal- ing, since it can reflect the idea that an individual might learn, might be reinforced, or might otherwise stabilize in the abstinent state as time progresses. There are though equally appealing alternatives which account for the data and which do not involve an individual changing over time. If, for example, each individual has a different predisposition or vulner- ability, and this remains with him or her unchanged as time passes, whether a relapse occurs under the vagaries of chance is dependent upon a mechanism which has no historical development, no past memory, and no future changing prognosis. Yet this equally will produce on average for a group of people an observed declining overall probability of relapse, as the more vulnerable succumb more quickly, leaving the tougher to relapse more slowly at a later time. The overall risk for the group thus appears to drop lower as time goes on and cannot be used to discriminate between these two models of process at the level of the individual.

The very simple group analysis for relapse risks described above can be extended in more interesting ways. The analysis of the MRFIT data in the paper referenced above looks behind the risk time-course and specifies a model which offers a more immediate understanding of a changing risk for an individual. The simple development which Fan provides is based on two unmeasured pressures, one to revert to smok- ing and one to regain abstinence, each of which decline over time, but not necessarily at the same rate of change, in a tightly specified way. By using information on relapse and secondary cessation it is possible to separate these two countervailing pressures; details are given in the referenced works.

If the likelihood that different individuals have different probabilities of relapse is taken seriously in these models, then a highly predictive model is one in which various risk factors which influence this proba- bility can be identified, so that for a given person at a given time the risk will be raised to one or lowered to zero; or, put more accurately and less demandingly, it will be shifted well away from the mean level of the whole group. In general, it must be said that risk models do not achieve this highly predictive status, and that risk factors are usually weak. Within the literature for each type of drug of addiction various competing factors make their appearance as candidates for bestowing predictive powers upon the models, some appearances brief and some more persistent. It is not the purpose of this chapter to review these factors, but to be content with generalities about their generally weak nature. Whether this lack of predictive power arises from the model itself, from the definitional difficulties involved, or from the phenomenon itself is a question that requires critical attention.

Characterizing the phenomenon of relapse

Survival curves are often criticized as not capturing the essence of the process of relapse but instead focusing on a very limiting definition of the first stage after treatment or cessation, that is, up to the first ingestion of the drug and ignoring subsequent changes—and it is clear that they do effectively take the view that 'after one drink, you're gone'. The alternative is to consider amending the definition of relapse in some way. The most evident way is to take not the first ingestion of the drug concerned, but to take the reaching of some threshold of consumption as determining the critical time-point at which relapse occurs. In fact the alcohol relapse curve just presented in Fig. 2.2 is constructed in this way, using a criterion of 3 months accumulated heavy or troubled drinking as the threshold. It might be thought that the entire process of relapse could be satisfactorily characterized by using a whole family of such thresholds to simultaneously identify the state of progression at any point. Initial attempts to use this blanket approach with this data set proved distinctly uninformative. It is, though, worth recording that instances of more successful use of this idea do exist: one such is an analysis of progressive relapse defined as the surpassing for several consecutive days of increasingly higher thresholds of troubled drinking (Drummond and Glautier 1994).

A more sophisticated approach is to build into the process the con-cept of a minor slip, as distinguished from a full-blown relapse (after Marlatt and Gordon 1985). Definitional difficulties aside, this must be a more promising direction in which to build. The problem is, though, one of complicating the identified course of the process by having multiple states, as opposed to just use or abstinence of a drug, by which to characterize it at any time-point.

The use of multiple states involves modelling a process by probabili-ties of transition not just from abstinence to use, but from any one state to any other, and back. In particular, therefore, such a conceptualization allows the study of secondary cessation transitions, secondary relapses, and so on: a multiplicity of entries into and departures from a given state as well as a multiplicity of states. Models of this extended nature generally come under the heading of 'event history' analysis.

An example of such an analysis can be taken from the same smoking treatment study as the first data set (due to Swan and Denk 1987), although it covers only a one-year period after treatment. Details of these results will not be presented here, except to note that the average rate of first relapse was approximately 4 per cent per month and of secondary cessation about 7 per cent per month. It is interesting to note that the researchers found no need to allow these probabilities of transition to vary directly with time: the observed decline in risk over time is accounted for by the individual differences concealed within these average rates, as was seen above.

In a model of this general nature the process is made individual-specific by identifying the relevant risk factors that distinguish one person from another: strain due to the type of occupation, parental smoking, gender, and nicotine consumption for example were identified in this study. Furthermore, risk factors can be incorporated which are associated with the individual's situation or disposition at the actual time of transition from one status to another: for instance the level of 'hassle' and the change in body-weight were found relevant. This latter set of risk factors, which change both over time and from one individual to the next, allow the characterization and tracking of the truly individual processes which give rise to the apparent process observed at the group level.

The price to be paid for such a detailed level of modeling is that the data required to estimate the parameters of risk have to be of high quality and must be collected at relevant and relatively frequent points throughout the period of study. It is perhaps the quality of data in the smoking field, in particular the easy measurement of consumption and the easily obtained quality of biological markers, that has encouraged these detailed studies.

REPEATED CESSATION AND RELAPSE

This last quoted study effectively abandons the restrictive approach of looking at simple treatment evaluation of a single episode. Once we move beyond the primary period of abstinence to looking at repeated cessation we have an immediate problem of attribution: can a second cessation be attributable to the initial treatment episode? And can a further treatment episode along with any subsequent abstinence be attributed indirectly to the initial treatment episode? The obverse of this particular coin is that in assessing a single treatment episode without reference to previous treatment episodes, let alone to spontaneous attempts to quit drug-taking, we are making a very strong statement about the modular nature of the process we are proposing.

If we do allow effects contingent upon a second episode of treatment to be in some sense attributed to the first, then with a little logic-chopping we can argue that only the first treatment ever should be awarded the responsibility for all later abstinence or relapse. More realistically, we would deduce that the treatment history to date must be included with the current treatment when we seek to attribute causation. In point of fact there appears to be some variability between different studies in showing an effect attributable to treatment history.

For longer-term studies looking at repeated cycles of abstinence and relapse, in view of the difficulties accompanying detailed event history analyses and in view of the limitations of survival analyses, it is not clear whether using the far cruder concept of simple prevalence at each of a series of time-points is a retrogressive or forward step. Fig. 2.4*a* and *b* are taken from an analysis of the Treatment Outcome Prospective Study (TOPS) data for cessation and relapse in drug addiction (Hubbard (ed.) 1989), and present such point-prevalences at a series of time-points both during treatment and after termination of treatment. The results of three treatment regimes, over a period of 5 years, for heroin addiction are shown in the figures.

Figures of this sort need to be treated with some circumspection when trying to make inferences about the immediate effect and its extended time course that result from a treatment episode, or inferences about the process of treatment and recovery. Although by using point prevalence of abstinence they are free from the complications of sustained abstinence definitions and from survival/risk interpretations, they display a further common difficulty in attributing causality.

By way of a simplistic demonstration, consider the following totally arbitrary situation in which a group of people use a drug—'use' being defined in any simple way as regular, or frequent, or whatever—but use it in an on—off fashion: that is, use and non-use for periods in no predictable pattern. There is then the possibility of falling prey to what one might call the coincident fallacy (there may be an existing proper nomenclature for the phenomenon to be described, here it will be termed the coincident fallacy). We might represent this pattern of behaviour in a simple way as a succession of boxes and dashes (here for ten people), as in Fig. 2.5*a*.

If then some of these periods of use are arbitrarily designated as ending in a treatment episode which has a null effect (represented by

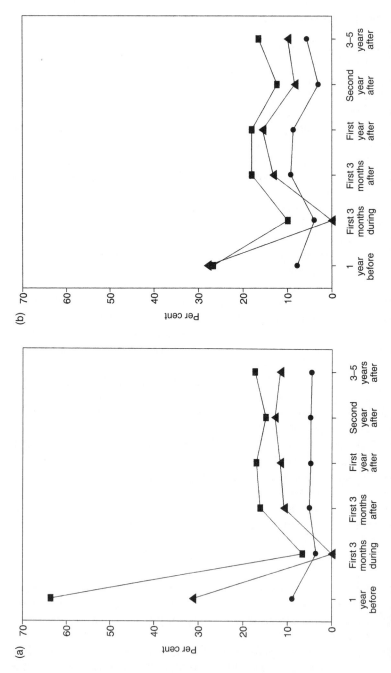

FIG. 2.4 (*a*) Changes in prevalence of regular heroin use (clients treated three months or longer); (*b*) Changes in prevalence of regular cocaine use (clients treated three months or longer). [(Taken from TOPS data, Hubbard (ed.) 1989.) The three regimes are represented by squares for Outpatient Methadone, triangles for Residential, and circles for Outpatient Drug-free.]

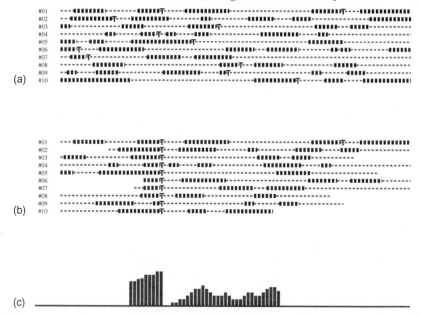

FIG. 2.5 (a) Random patterns of drug use for ten subjects across time; (b) aligned random patterns of heroin use (see text); (c) prevalence for aligned random patterns (see text).(Taken from TOPS data, Hubbard (ed.) 1989.)

a letter T in the figure), assuming nothing more than that a random selection of the abstinences immediately follow an arbitrarily designated point called 'treatment' which does not alter or disturb the existing pattern, we have a process with a null treatment effect introduced at random points. The purely random nature of cessation and relapse and its lack of association with 'treatment' must be emphasized in this behaviour pattern. However, simply by aligning all the treatment points at the same point in time on a second figure as in Fig. 2.5*b*, as one effectively does in an analysis which is based on measuring time beyond that treatment point, it is easy to see that on a prevalence chart (Fig. 2.5*c*) the effect is to produce a dramatic fall following treatment and a subsequent slow rise back to the original levels—and in some cases to fluctuating levels—before stabilizing.

It is not enough, therefore, to note that there is a drop in prevalence in order to argue that treatment has been effective: in the above figures treatment had no impact on the patterns of use and abstinence. To assess whether treatment has been effective it is necessary to compare the post-treatment stable level with the stable level which was obtained some time before the treatment alignment point. Equivalently, one might compare the length of the immediately following period of abstinence, or subsequent periods of abstinence, relative to lengths of periods of use with those before treatment though this latter information is usually difficult to obtain.

It is not intended to imply that this is what is happening in the TOPS data sets, where the prevalence levels may well be lower after treatment. Rather it is to make the general point that allowance must be made for this fallacy when analysing any results of this kind. At the very least it must be observed that processes of change which are apparent at a system or group level might correspond to a very different process in operation within an individual. At worst an observed post-treatment improvement might correspond to no process of change at all within the individual, as in this example. Again it seems that once we move to studying repeated periods of abstinence and use, especially over a long term, the role attributed to treatment in causing them is easily distorted.

In all this the question of 'spontaneous' cessation or more precisely cessation without an immediately preceding episode of formal treatment, has been deliberately skirted. This is undoubtedly an important phenomenon in all fields of addiction as is testified by the considerable literature which exists on the subject (see for example Smart 1976; Tuchfeld 1984). Smoking is typically the field in which it appears that most attempts to quit are not related to a treatment episode, as evidenced by a spontaneous cessation prevalence of around 40 per cent and a very small number of people who are formally treated. Clearly the questions associated with specific attribution of causality are different in the absence of treatment. There is almost certainly less reason under these circumstances to study a single cycle of cessation and relapse, and rather more reason for paying attention to the continuity of effect across such attempts. It is this concept of continuity through all attempts, spontaneous or not, to which we now turn.

LIFE-COURSE AND CAREER

Let us now look through the other end of the telescope, that is, to expand the time-window and to stand back far enough from the detail of events to take in if not the whole of a lifespan at least a large slice of it. It is in many ways an attractive argument that the relevance of the concept of a treatment episode and its associated outcome now disappears. The very first episode of treatment may be a significant milestone in the life-history of the client, but working in this time-scale the outcome of that or any other treatment episode must more properly be thought of as the whole of the succeeding life course, rather than any particular point along the way.

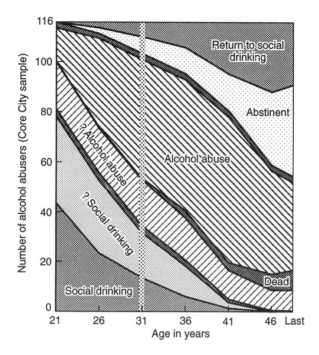

FIG. 2.6 Composite of alcohol use and abuse among the 116 Core City men ever classified as alcohol abusers. The stippled area refers to the proportion drinking asymptomatically; lighter stippling indicates diagnostic uncertainty. Diagonal lines reflect men with four or more symptoms of alcohol abuse; widely spaced diagonal lines indicate diagnostic uncertainty. The crosshatched line at age 31 is intended to accentuate differences in age of onset of alcohol abuse in the different samples in this and the following figures. (From Vaillant 1983.)

If one were to put to one side for a moment the treatment/outcome framework of analysis and look instead at the passage of time, the use of detailed models of the processes at work becomes extremely difficult, partly because of the complexity likely to be demanded of such a model if it is to have any explanatory power, and partly because of the level of data collection that is required to identify the parameters of such a model. Data collection at points separated by a 5-year interval, for instance, would be quite a luxury to enjoy. Our understanding of the processes taking place must come from a very much more descriptive approach, at a much coarser level both of categorization of status within the processes and of the time units used to chart it.

In *The natural history of alcoholism* (1983) Vaillant presents a fascinating summary chart, which is reproduced here as Fig. 2.6, of a birth cohort of 116 'Core City men' who at some point were categorized as 'abusing alcohol'. The indication of a process at work is suggested by the vertical ordering of the categories showing stages of development from social drinking, through alcohol abuse to abstinence, and the possible return to social drinking.

Thus we are led to watch, as we move through the years, across the figure, men being recruited from social drinker into the 'sometime alcohol abuser' category: and for each year the men above this line of passage become alcohol abusers who may move back and forth between abstinence, social drinking, and alcohol abuse again.

There are two pieces of information welded together in this figure. The first can be seen if we look at the passage from social drinking to alcohol abuse (at the bottom of the diagram), the numbers recruited into abuse naturally increase with time, but so does the rate at which this is happening gradually increase with age throughout the span of the figure: and this is not counter-intuitive. A little rough calculation shows that this is so whether we use the loose or more strict definition of social drinking indicated in the diagram.

Above that line of passage from social drinking to alcohol abuse we have a second set of information: the percentage of people—or equivalently of time spent—in various states, by one-time alcohol abusers. Even if we allow for the swelling numbers of alcohol abusers, the *percentage* of people from the group in the recovery categories of abstinence and social drinking increases as the cohort ages. Indeed the data seem remarkable, to someone dealing mostly with clinic samples, for the proportion of people at any time in the category of 'returned to social drinking'. As Vaillant has pointed out, this chart pertains to people who have been observed from their first episode of alcohol abuse onwards, and this is not a clinic sample. It is easy to see that any tendency for entrenchment in alcohol abuse to be accompanied by increased numbers of appearances at alcoholism clinics means that clinic samples will always be automatically self-weighted towards the worst clinic attenders.

By way of contrast Fig. 2.7 presents a life-chart drawn up from the Addiction Research Unit's long-term follow-up study of clinic attenders, although it presents information of a slightly different nature. The information is taken from a paper on a 20-year follow-up of 100 male alcoholics attending an alcoholism clinic in 1968/9. Here the horizontal axis indicates years elapsed since the indexing treatment episode (which was often not their first episode), rather than chronological age. The amount of time spent by the group as a whole in drinking or abstinence is shown on the vertical axis in units of person-months, though the data were collected in considerably coarser units than this. Thus the bottom area indicates time spent in abstinence or light social drinking, this latter

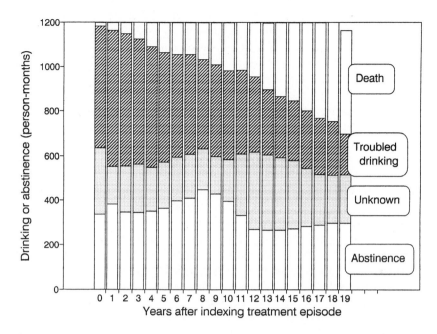

FIG. 2.7 Life chart over 20 years of 100 male alcoholics.

category being very tightly defined. The area above it shows time spent in an unknown fashion and arises only in small part from loss of information due to attrition of the sample; mostly it arises because the behaviours are self-reported, and, therefore a death prior to a follow-up interview—which were here 10 years apart—deprives us of all information on the elapsed period. The top category represents time lost to the cohort through death; and the remaining category, represents time spent in troubled drinking, defined either by consumption levels or alcohol-related physical symptoms.

It would be tempting to argue that the level of abstinent time remains more or less constant within the group as a whole, and that troubled drinking gives way only to death. Of course we cannot make this assertion, since this form of presentation gives no indication of which individual is behaving in the described fashion, or to which behavioural category he might next move. At this level of description any suggestion of following individual time-courses is lost; we are left with the possibility of comparing different cohorts or different sub-groups of the same cohort. In a previous publication (Taylor *et al.* 1986) the authors tried to use cluster analysis to identify behaviourally different groups within the cohort, at least in relation to dependence, drinking levels, and physical damage. Through their contrasting life-charts this approach can provide information on the different life-courses contained within the overall cohort. In these data we have sought to see whether there is a divergence of courses between the important categories of levels of alcohol dependence. In fact, quoting here some provisional figures, subsequent analysis of this set of data for the 20-year follow-up does show a significantly greater excess of mortality amongst people classified as severely dependent at the indexing treatment episode when compared with those classified as only moderately dependent. The life-chart (not presented here) also shows death eating into the severely dependent group more heavily at the expense of time spent in troubled drinking, but this may not prove to be a statistically significant difference.

Other studies have developed this idea. Stimson and Oppenheimer (Stimson and Ogborne 1970) have tried to identify distinct life-styles of heroin addicts, based on cluster analysis. Work in progress at the National Addiction Centre is currently analysing a 20-year follow-up in terms of these sub-groups to look for diverging processes of development.

Returning for a moment to the question of treatment, which does not appear in these life-charts, it would seem to me that unless it can firmly demonstrated that the effect of treatment at any one time is independent of previous treatment—a proposition which few would adopt a priori as their most favoured position—then the role of individual treatment episodes falls away, and instead a unified treatment history has to be fundamentally woven into the processes we wish to characterize. We need in fact to take a whole treatment career, as Griffith Edwards (1984) calls it, as one career amongst others such as the social career and the drinking career, and seek to describe how it interweaves not only with these other aspects of overall career, but also with the natural history of the biological processes which might underly the time-course of addiction.

One treatment episode though certainly does warrant special attention, and that is the first-ever treatment. It would be justifiable to single this out simply because if one were to characterize an addiction career by important milestones throughout its course, this first overt appeal for help in ceasing to use drugs, even if preceded by 'spontaneous' attempts, must be pre-eminent. Oppenheimer and colleagues (Oppenheimer *et al.* 1988) have reported a study of addicts who are new to treatment— that is those who have been interviewed at their first treatment episode. Fig. 2.8 displays data taken from their study which relates the important milestones of age at first drug use, first opiate use, first injection, and first treatment. These are crude markers. It would perhaps be better to look at when drug use became regular, rather than at the occasion of first use. However, defining regular use is difficult and to pin-point a

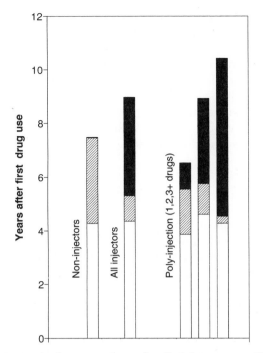

FIG. 2.8 Milestones in drug use—lags after first drug use: until first opiate use (open column); until first injection (hatched column), and until first treatment (black column).

particular associated age even more difficult. Taking the point of first use, which is likely to be more memorable in people's minds, probably has the advantage of a being more reliable and clear-cut measure.

In fact this figure shows these milestones for sub-groups of the overall sample, and shows them as lags after first drug use, which itself was relatively uniform across these groupings: respectively from bottom to top, lag to first opiate use, lag to first injection, and lag to coming for treatment. The pattern which emerges is that those who never turn to injecting (first column) come in for treatment first and those who do turn to injecting (second column) take longer. The third to fifth columns are a breakdown of those who inject, classified by whether they have injected only one drug (almost always heroin), or have at some point injected a second drug, or three or more; this might crudely be expected to indicate how bad an injection habit they have. As can be seen, on this interpretation, whatever the process is which is at work in bringing people into treatment, it needs to account for the fact that those with the worst habit have taken longest to come in for treatment.

When looking to see how this progressive recruitment pattern differs between various other groupings in the sample, one might anticipate that it would differ for groups with differences in their drug abuse patterns; but what of differences between biological and social factors such as sex, criminal history before drug use, level of educational attainment, and whether they live alone or with a partner or with another addict? No differences in any of these sub-groupings were found, although there was some suggestion that those with children, those in full-time employ, and those homeless stayed out longest.

CONCLUSIONS

By way of conclusion, it should be re-iterated that no attempt has been made here to give a comprehensive coverage of models of addiction processes; on the contrary, there has been a highly selective choice of strategies for constructing data-based models. Rather than conclude with a résumé of how one might model the time-course of an addiction career, instead we will conclude by raising the stakes, so to speak, by posing a yet more difficult question. Why do we measure the time-course in units of time? And is this use of the obvious chronological units the most sensible choice? If, for example, it can be suggested that in a smoking career the risk of lung cancer relates to the total number of cigarettes smoked, life-long, might it not be more useful to base our view of progression not on units of time but on units of total drug flow? Or, if we baulk at the idea of time standing still during periods of abstinence, why not at least think of time slowing in those periods and accelerating during drug taking? A major conceptual re-thinking is not being suggested here, but merely an expression of irritation and concern that our characterizing the course of events so often has the same units measured along the horizontal axis. This chapter, though, is not an appropriate forum in which to take up these challenges.

REFERENCES

Bradley, B. P. (1989). In *Relapse and addictive behaviour* (ed. M. Gossop), pp. 73–85. Routledge, London.

Drummond, C. D. and Glautier, S. (1994). A controlled trial of cue exposure treatment in alcohol dependence II: treatment outcome. *Journal of Consulting and Clinical Psychology*. (In press.)

Edwards, G. (1984). Drinking in longitudinal perspective: career and natural history. *British Journal of Addiction*, **79**, 175–83.

Fan, D. P. (1985). Ideodynamic predictions for the evolution of habits. *Journal of Mathematical Sociology*, **11**, 265–81.

Fan, D. P. and Elketroussi, M. (1989). Mathematical model for addiction: application to Multiple Risk Factor Intervention Trial data for smoking. *Journal of Consulting and Clinical Psychology*, **57**, 456–9.

Gossop, M., Green, L., Phillips, G., and Bradley, B. P. (1989). Lapse, relapse and survival among opiate addicts after treatment: a prospective follow-up study. *British Journal of Psychiatry*, **154**, 348–53.

Hubbard, R. L. (ed.) (1989). *Drug abuse treatment: a national study of effectiveness*. University of North Carolina Press, Chapel Hill.

Marlatt, G. A. and Gordon, J. R. (ed.) (1985). *Relapse prevention: maintenance strategies in the treatment of addictive behaviour*. Guilford Press, New York.

Oppenheimer, E., Sheehan, M., and Taylor, C. (1988). Letting the clients speak: drug misusers and the process of help seeking. *British Journal of Addiction*, **83**, 635–47.

Smart, R. G. (1976). Spontaneous recovery in alcoholics: a review and analysis of the available literature. *Drug and Alcohol Dependence*, **1**, 227–85.

Stimson, G. V. and Ogborne, A. (1970). Survey of a representative sample of addicts prescribed heroin at London clinics. *Bulletin on Narcotics*, **22**, 13–22.

Swan, G. E. and Denk, C. E. (1987). Dynamic models for the maintenance of smoking cessation: event history analysis of late relapse. *Journal of Behavioural Medicine*, **10**, 527–54.

Taylor, C., Brown, D., Duckitt, A., Edwards, G., Oppenheimer, E., and Sheehan, M. (1985). Patterns of outcome: drinking histories over 10 years among a group of alcoholics. *British Journal of Addiction*, **80**, 45–50.

Taylor, C., Brown, D., Duckitt, A., Edwards, G., Oppenheimer, E., and Sheehan, M. (1986). Alcoholism and the patterning of outcome: a multivariate analysis. *British Journal of Addiction*, **81**, 815–23.

Tuchfeld, B. S. (1981). Spontaneous remission in alcoholics: empirical observations an theoretical implications. *Quarterly Journal of Studies on Alcohol*, **42**, 626–41.

Vaillant, G. (1983). *The natural history of alcoholism*. Harvard University Press, Cambridge, Massachusetts.

3

The changing pharmacology of addiction

DAVID NUTT

INTRODUCTION

To a considerable extent this book discusses change processes within a psychological perspective, and the value of the insights which come from that view is undoubted. However, in discussing change within the very broad context of addiction it would be a mistake to ignore the physical dimensions. Indeed, arguably the greatest advance in our understanding of the processes of addiction has been the discovery that addictive drugs have a discrete pharmacology. It is now possible to explain the actions of most abused agents in terms of interactions with specific neurochemical processes in the brain. These are usually interactions with specific receptors but sometimes can be with transport proteins or enzymes. It is possible to classify addictive drugs in terms of their pharmacology as shown in Table 3.1.

A number of important concepts emerge from a knowledge of the pharmacology of addictive agents, these are discussed in the context of the critical issues in drug addiction; tolerance, dependence, withdrawal, and abuse potential. Before that it is useful to outline briefly a few relevant pharmacological constructs that contribute to our understanding of these processes.

AGONISM AND ANTAGONISM

Most of the addictive agents for which a pharmacology has been established behave as agonists, which means that they mimic the actions of an endogenous transmitter system. Thus heroin acts at receptors for which the endogenous mediators are the endorphin or enkephalin

TABLE 3.1 *Classification of addictive drugs in terms of their pharmacology*

Drug class	Site and type of action
Opioid	mu opioid receptors
Stimulants	
cocaine	monoamine esp. dopamine uptake blockade
amphetamine	monoamine release
nicotine	dopamine release
MDMA (ecstasy)	? 5-HT release
Hallucinogens	
LSD	? $5\text{-}HT_2$ receptors
phencyclidine	excitatory amino acid (EAA) blockade
ketamine	EAA blockade
Sedatives	
barbiturates	GABA-A receptor stimulation, EAA block
alcohol(s)	GABA-A receptor stimulation, EAA block
benzodiazepines	benzodiazepine/GABA-A receptor
Cannabis	receptors
Solvents	? EAA block
Caffeine	? adenosine receptor blockade

peptides. Cocaine and amphetamines act as indirect dopamine agonists by increasing synaptic availability of this transmitter. As dopamine release generally results in activation this probably explains the stimulant actions of these drugs. In contrast, the benzodiazepines and barbiturates act by increasing the efficacy of the natural transmitter gamma-aminobutyric acid (GABA). As GABA is the major inhibitory transmitter in the brain these drugs tend to be sedating.

Antagonists are drugs which block the actions of agonists but which have no intrinsic actions at their binding sites. Some abused drugs are antagonists, particularly of the recently discovered excitatory amino acid (EAA) receptors. It seems likely that the dissociative states produced by phencyclidine, ketamine, barbiturates, and alcohol are all mediated by a blockade of one or more of the three major types of EAA receptor. Since these receptors are responsible for the relaying of primary sensory information into the brain their interruption leads to a functional sensory denervation−dissociation. Their pleasurable qualities may be a result of this pharmacological detachment from the real world.

AFFINITY AND EFFICACY

Affinity is a measure that describes the avidity with which a drug (sometimes called a ligand) binds to its site of action, usually a receptor or enzyme. The higher the affinity of a drug the less is required to occupy enough receptors to produce a given effect. Thus, once allowance is made for pharmacokinetic variables, such as absorption and metabolism, the higher the affinity of an abused drug the less that has to be taken to produce a rewarding effect. Thus the difference in doses of opioids used by addicts is determined largely by the relative affinities of the various compounds for the mu opioid receptor.

The efficacy of an agonist drug is a measure of the maximal response that it can produce. A related construct is the percentage of receptors needed to be occupied by an agonist to produce a given effect. As a concept it can only be applied to directly acting agonists such as the opioids and the drugs that bind to the GABA-A receptor complex. The opioids provide the most extensive characterization of efficacy, as a range of compounds have been synthesized that span the spectrum from full agonist through partial agonists to antagonists (Table 3.2). The agonist opioids heroin, morphine, and methadone have roughly similar efficacies. Partial agonists, such as buprenorphine or nalbuphine, never produce the same maximal effect as full agonists even at receptor saturation. The maximal effects of partial agonists always come at full receptor occupation and can vary from nearly those of full agonists to so very little that they resemble antagonists. Moreover, when given in combination with an agonist they antagonize its action in a dose-related fashion; hence they are sometimes called agonist-antagonists. Antagonists by definition have zero efficacy, that is, they have no intrinsic effects even at receptor saturation, although they may have profound actions due to their blockade of ongoing agonist activity.

A full spectrum of efficacy from agonists through partial agonists to antagonists has also been discovered for both GABA-A and benzodiazepine receptors. Relatively little work has been done with either full or partial agonists that act at the GABA receptor. One compound,

TABLE 3.2 *The opioid efficacy spectrum*

Agonist	Partial agonist	Antagonist
Morphine	buprenorphine > nalbuphine	naloxone
Heroin		naltrexone
Methadone		

TABLE 3.3 *The spectrum of efficacy at the benzodiazepine receptor*

Agonist	Partial agonist	Antagonist	Partial inverse agonist	Inverse agonist
Diazepam	bretazenil	flumazenil	FG 7142	DMCM
Lorazepam	abecarnil	ZK 93426	sarazenil	β-CCCM
Temazepam				
Triazolam				
Alprazolam				
Oxazepam				
etc				

THIP, a full agonist with anticonvulsant properties, was given to a few volunteers but produced bizarre motor effects and so its development was stopped. Much more is known about the range of compounds acting at the benzodiazepine receptor (reviewed by Nutt 1990*a*). The traditional benzodiazepines, such as diazepam and lorazepam, act as full agonists, producing maximal effects at between 30–50 per cent of receptor occupancy depending on the test. These actions are fully blocked by antagonists such as flumazenil (see Table 2.3). Recently a series of different partial agonists have been discovered. These have a lower efficacy, often requiring maximal receptor occupancy to produce an effect. As with the opioid partial agonists these compounds are relatively free of unwanted actions; they produce little ataxia and sedation and show less potentiation of the effects of alcohol or other sedatives. In addition, benzodiazepine receptor partial agonists will block some actions of full agonists, particularly sedation.

The benzodiazepine receptor is unusual in that it also binds compounds which have the opposite actions to classic benzodiazepine agonists. These ligands are called inverse agonists and are anxiogenic and proconvulsant. We know they act at the same receptor site as the agonists because their actions are blocked by antagonists. The discovery of the bidirectional nature of the benzodiazepine receptor makes it hard to determine their role in the brain, since they may mediate anxiety and arousal as well as anxiolysis and inhibition. Until the endogenous ligand for the benzodiazepine receptor is found this question will remain unresolved. However, alterations in the function of the benzodiazepine receptor have been suggested to play a part in benzodiazepine tolerance and withdrawal as well as in some anxiety states (see below and Nutt 1990*b*).

THE FOUR PILLARS OF ADDICTION: TOLERANCE, DEPENDENCE, WITHDRAWAL, AND ABUSE POTENTIAL

These four interlinked constructs were seen, until the emergence of HIV, as the central issues in opioid addiction and still are for most other abused drugs. The quartet form a self-reinforcing circuit where tolerance can lead to dose escalation, and thus to greater withdrawal (physical dependence), which in turn encourages maintenance dosing. It is important to be aware that although often interlinked these are discrete phenomena which can sometimes be differentiated; for instance dependence from abuse potential. A good example of physical dependence unrelated to abuse is that which may be produced iatrogenically by the chronic prescription of benzodiazepines. Similarly, many patients with chronic pain become dependent on opioids but never abuse them. An example of abuse without dependence may be the use of lysergic acid diethylamide (LSD) and the bingeing intake of alcohol characteristic of young drinkers.

The mechanisms of tolerance, withdrawal, and abuse potential are generally better understood than those of psychological dependence. This is because animal models of dependence are less satisfactory and because as a construct it probably encompasses more than one variable.

Tolerance

Tolerance is a process by which a living system attenuates the actions of applied agents such as drugs. This may occur at a number of levels (Table 3.4). Conditioned opponent processes are generated by organisms in an attempt to offset the maladaptive consequences of addictive (or other) agents and are conditioned by situational cues relating to drug use (for example a bar for alcoholics). Thus for sedating drugs and the opioids they are aspects of arousal, such as tachycardia and increased alertness. These processes can be demonstrated by administering placebo

TABLE 3.4 *Levels of tolerance*

Site	Process
Whole animal	conditioned opponent processes
Gut	reduced absorption
Liver/kidney	increased metabolism/clearance
Brain	compensatory (extrinsic) adaptation
Neurone	receptor (intrinsic) adaptation

TABLE 3.5 *Adaptive processes (where known)*

Drug class	Changes in brain
Opioids	receptor desensitization (?phosphorylation) inc. calcium channels
Stimulants	increased dopamine release,? inc. receptors
Barbiturates	dec. GABA function, inc. EAA receptors
Alcohol	dec. GABA function, ? inc. inverse agonist inc. EAA receptors, inc. calcium channels dec α_2-adrenoceptors
Benzodiazepines	receptor shift in inverse agonist direction ? inc. inverse agonist
LSD	? receptor down-regulation

dec., decreased; inc., increased.

when drug is expected. In some cases conditioned opponent responses may be sufficiently powerful to produce a withdrawal-like state. It is thought that this is also an important component of craving. Conversely unexpected deaths due to opioid use in new environments has been ascribed to a deficit in such adaptive processes leading to functional overdose (see Siegel 1976, 1984).

Pharmacokinetic factors may, in theory, contribute to tolerance to a range of drugs. They include alterations in absorption rate as well as increased metabolism and clearance. In practice there is not a great deal of evidence to suggest that these are major variables although delayed absorption of alcohol in chronic alcoholics has been reported. It is likely that the barbiturates, by inducing liver enzymes, contribute to their own metabolism (Goodman and Gilman 1985), which emphasizes the distinction between the barbiturates and the benzodiazepines.

The most studied forms of adaptation are those which are used by the end organ, the brain. I have classified these into extrinsic and intrinsic processes to emphasize the site of the adaptation. Intrinsic processes are those which are directly related to the site of action of the abused drug. The determinants of opioid tolerance are beginning to be understood. It is thought that this is due to a reduction in receptor number or a desensitization of function due to receptor phosphorylation or lack of access to second messenger proteins (Table 2.5) (see Kennedy and Henderson 1991). The efficacy of the opioid has a major bearing on the degree of tolerance production, with partial agonists producing a more rapid loss of their actions than is seen with full agonists. In this regard opioid tolerance is the direct opposite of benzodiazepine tolerance (see below). It seems likely that tolerance plays an important role in the action of maintenance therapies such as methadone. Prolonged exposure to this full agonist will lead to sufficient tolerance to negate the reinforcing actions of any illicitly-used opioid (a process known as cross-tolerance).

Tolerance to the benzodiazepines seems to involve an alteration in the spectrum of receptor function between agonist and inverse agonist. Thus the 'setpoint' (the neutral position in the middle of the spectrum) is moved, as manifest by agonists becoming less efficacious and antagonists behaving like weak inverse agonists (see Nutt 1990*b*). The ability of benzodiazepine receptor ligands to produce this shift in setpoint seems to be directly related to their intrinsic efficacy, with full agonists being the most active and partial agonists showing less, or no propensity to shift the 'setpoint' (Hernandez *et al.* 1989; Moreau *et al.* 1990). This has been well demonstrated in preclinical studies, and there is a smattering of clinical evidence that the same may be true in patients when partial agonists are used to treat epilepsy (see Haigh and Feely 1988).

It seems likely that a similar change in benzodiazepine receptor function may account for some of the tolerance to alcohol. However, this is unlikely to be the whole story as very recent evidence points to alterations in EAA receptor functions as also contributing to alcohol tolerance. A number of groups have described upregulation of NMDA (*N*-methyl-D-aspartate) receptor number following chronic alcohol exposure, presumably in an attempt to offset the depressant actions of the drug (reviewed by Glue and Nutt 1990).

Extrinsic processes may be parallel or sequential to the system that is the site of action of the drug. Thus in the case of the benzodiazepines compensatory upregulation of noradrenaline and 5-HT function may occur to offset the increased inhibition caused by enhanced GABA function. Removal of the elevated tone results in a relative excess of these monoamine transmitters which causes some of the symptoms of withdrawal (see Nutt 1990*b*). A similar situation applies to the opioids. Acutely they inhibit central noradrenergic neurones, tolerance occurs to this action, so in withdrawal these neurones are overactive (see below).

It is important to realize that not all addictive drugs uniformly produce tolerance. Stimulants, in particular cocaine, may produce the opposite effects of sensitization (kindling), in which some of the behavioural actions of the drug increase rather than decrease over time. There is some animal evidence that suggests sensitization to stimulants is in part due to higher brain levels following chronic administration, although receptor upregulation may also play a part. Loss of tolerance is also seen in end-stage alcoholism, probably due to brain and liver damage.

Dependence

Similar pharmacological factors as discussed for tolerance also underly dependence, thus the degree of tolerance is often an indication of the extent of dependence. Important variables are the duration of treatment and the efficacy of the drug used. The role of drugs with reduced efficacy—partial agonists—and antagonists in treating dependence is just beginning to be evaluated.

In the case of the opioids it has been suggested that the partial mu agonists may have significant potential as treatments for opioid abuse. The rationale for this is the ability of partial agonists to attenuate the actions of full agonists and yet have some reinforcing activity. An addict treated with a partial agonist will get less pleasure from any subsequent use of a full agonist. If the partial agonist has particularly high affinity for the mu receptor then complete blockade of reinforcement can be produced. The value of partial agonists producing some reinforcement is that they do not lead to the feelings of dysphoria and even depression that the long-acting antagonists such as naltrexone often produce (see below). Additionally, they give something of a 'buzz' each time they are given which helps encourage compliance. Furthermore, transition from street drugs (agonists) to partial agonists is easier to achieve than transfer to antagonists with their great propensity to precipitate withdrawal. Another important benefit of opioid partial agonists is that they are safer than full agonists. As a direct consequence of their having a lower efficacy they cause less respiratory depression, especially in overdose (see Jasinski *et al.* 1978).

The ideal characteristics of a partial agonist for the treatment of opioid addiction are high affinity (to fully block any agonist), long half-life (to minimize frequency of dosing), and adequate agonism to maximize compliance. Currently buprenorphine is the most promising candidate. It has been shown to block the actions of opioid agonists (Jasinski *et al.* 1978), to substitute for morphine without precipitation of withdrawal, and to be somewhat reinforcing, having a maximal effect about equal to that of 30 mg methadone (Strain *et al.* 1992). Large trials of buprenorphine in addicts are currently underway in the USA, since the National Institute of Drug Abuse aims to have it available as an alternative to methadone within a few years.

By analogy with the situation with the opioids it is possible that benzodiazepine receptor partial agonists may also have therapeutic potential, especially in the treatment of benzodiazepine dependence. As yet it is not known whether benzodiazepine partial agonists will block the actions of full agonists in man or whether they will precipitate withdrawal from full agonists. If, as hoped, they turn out to be free from dependence/withdrawal potential these partial agonists may re-surrect the concept of long-term benzodiazepine therapy, which for full agonists is not currently recommended by the Committee on Safety of Medicines.

Another approach to drug dependence is the use of selective anta-gonists. For instance, in the case of the benzodiazepines, flumazenil, which has recently become licensed for use in anaesthesia to reverse benzodiazepine sedation. Animal studies have revealed it to have the unexpected property of reducing dependence if given concurrently with agonists (Gallager *et al*. 1986) or even during withdrawal (Nutt and Costello 1988). It is currently being tried in patients with protracted withdrawal states and in dependent subjects prior to dose tapering. Therapeutically, there might be some use for a selective antagonist of the barbiturates, although the recent discovery of their other site of action at EAA receptors makes this prospect rather remote.

Opioid antagonists have been shown, like flumazenil, to reduce the degree of dependence on opioids in animals. Thus monkeys given nal-oxone at intervals during exposure to morphine showed less dependence on spontaneous withdrawal (Krystal *et al*. 1989). It would be interesting to see if a similar phenomenon could be demonstrated in humans for it might assist the detoxification process. Perhaps the practice of rapid detoxification from opioids using naltrexone/clonidine/benzodiazepine combinations is to some extent utilizing the same concept. Antagonists can also be used to help determine the degree of dependence on opioids; the greater the degree of dependence the greater the withdrawal state precipitated by the antagonist (Jaskinski *et al*. 1967).

A great deal of effort is currently being expended in the search for treatments of cocaine dependence (see Gawin 1991). Some have suggested that mazindol, another uptake blocker, might be such a drug, although detailed interaction studies have not yet been performed. Alternatively, if cocaine releases dopamine would dopamine receptor antagonists be of use? Some reports have suggested they might, for instance depot fluphenazine reduced cocaine use in one study. Recent monkey and rat investigations have demonstrated that the opioid buprenorphine exerts a powerful blockade of cocaine reinforcement (Mello *et al*. 1989). Why buprenorphine should have this ability is the subject of much current research, and whether it should be prescribed for cocaine addicts is a matter of some debate at present (Kosten *et al*. 1989) although the concept has been patented!

Withdrawal

This phenomenon is usually construed as the expression of those processes underlying tolerance revealed by the removal of the addictive
agent from the body. This is likely to be largely correct although, at least
in the case of alcohol, there is evidence that tolerance and withdrawal
can be differentially modified pharmacologically (reviewed in Nutt and
Glue 1986). In general, withdrawal from sedating agents produces a
state of increased excitability, whereas that from stimulants often has
lethargy as a cardinal feature.

The adaptive processes that may explain withdrawal are listed in
Table 2.5. It can be seen that several of the drugs produce similar changes
in the brain. Thus alcohol, opioids, and perhaps the barbiturates, but
not the benzodiazepines, have been shown to increase the number of
calcium channels (reviewed in Silverstone and Grahame-Smith 1992).
This increase in calcium channel number probably contributes directly
to the hyperexcitability seen in withdrawal from these drugs as it facilitates greater calcium influx into neurones. Support for this contention
is given by the observed beneficial effect of calcium channel antagonists
in animal models, although this needs confirmation in humans. An
important consequence of increased calcium influx is that it can cause
neuronal death and this may be a factor in alcoholic brain damage.
If so it would argue that alcohol withdrawal is itself a danger to the
patient and so should be actively treated. Another factor that contributes
to calcium influx in alcohol withdrawal is the upregulation of NMDA
receptors mentioned above. Excessive NMDA activity produces brain
excitability leading to anxiety, seizures, and increased calcium influx
(see Glue and Nutt 1990). There is some suggestion that NMDA function
is increased by chronic opioid use so it would be of interest to investigate
whether opioid withdrawal also leads to greater calcium influx and cell
damage.

Another common factor in withdrawal from sedating drugs is that
of noradrenergic overactivity, as demonstrated by increased central
and peripheral release of noradrenaline and its metabolites. It appears
that this is mediated by different mechanisms. In the case of the opioids
the loss of inhibitor tone is, in part, the result of a compensatory build
up of the second messenger cyclic AMP, although other more directly
receptor-linked mechanisms also play a part (see Kennedy and Henderson
1991). With alcohol there appears to be a loss, or subsensitivity of the
inhibitoryα_2-adrenoceptors that autoregulate noradrenergic neuronal activity (Nutt *et al.* 1988). In withdrawal from the benzodiazepines it seems
that decreased GABA-A mediated inhibition is to blame, which also
contributes to alcohol withdrawal (see Glue and Nutt 1990). Whatever

the explanation the increased noradrenergic activation can be suppressed by clonidine and related drugs which, because they act as agonists at the inhibitory α_2-adrenoceptors, inhibit neuronal activity (Aghajanian 1978).

Abuse liability

The factors which determine abuse liability are listed in Table 2.6. It is apparent that both pharmacokinetic and pharmacodynamic factors are important. The rate at which a drug enters the brain seems to markedly affect its abuse potential, the faster the better. For instance, the lipophilic benzodiazepine diazepam enters very quickly and has a greater street value than the much slower onset benzodiazepine oxazepam, which would appear to have little or no abuse liability (Griffiths *et al*. 1984). Addicts have developed a range of techniques for accelerating the access of drug to brain. The most obvious are intravenous injections and the making of volatile free-base forms of cocaine and amphetamine that can be smoked. The lungs offer a remarkable surface area for drug absorption, so plasma levels of inhaled drugs peak almost as fast as when they are taken intravenously. This fact helps to explain the highly addictive nature of nicotine.

Pharmacodynamic factors relate to the intrinsic actions of the drugs. Here again efficacy becomes a critical variable, the more efficacious the drug the more addictive it is. A good example is the well-recognized difference in the abuse potential of the barbiturates and the benzodiazepines (Griffiths *et al*. 1980). This is mirrored by the significantly greater efficacy of the barbiturates in terms of their ability to augment the actions of GABA. Partial agonist benzodiazepines should, therefore,

TABLE 3.6 *Determinants of abuse liability*

1. **Reinforcing potential**
    (a) *Pharmacokinetics*—Rate of entry into brain
        route: smoke = i.v. > nasal > oral
        drug factors: lipophilicity, solubility

    (b) *Pharmacodynamics*—Actions in brain
        high efficacy, e.g. barbiturates > benzodiazepines
            opioid full agonists > partial agonists
        fast onset and offset of receptor interactions

2. **Availability**
    better = more abuse

have no abuse potential, a supposition confirmed by studies which show that animals will not work to obtain them, that is they are not reinforcing.

Similar findings have been established for the opioids where both animal and human experiments have revealed a roughly proportional relationship between efficacy and reinforcement. Thus partial agonists are less pleasurable and have a lower street value. Nalbuphine appears to be at the threshold of reinforcing actions and drugs with a lower efficacy should have no abuse potential. Unfortunately, they are also unlikely to be analgesic. In theory it should be possible to block the reinforcing actions of high efficacy opioids by pretreatment with partial agonists. This has been established in animal work and new studies with buprenorphine have revealed that a similar effect can be produced in man (Strain *et al*. 1992).

Of course it is also possible to block the effects of those addictive drugs which act as agonists by the administration of antagonists with a greater affinity for the same receptors. Thus naloxone or naltrexone are potent mu antagonists which prevent the pleasurable actions of opioids (see Jasinski *et al*. 1978). Antagonists have uses that extend beyond pharmacologically defining the receptor-specific actions of abused drugs. They can be used in several ways to help prevent or to treat drug abuse. A well-established role is in the maintenance of abstinence. The best example of this is naltrexone in opioid addicts. This is a potent and long-acting antagonist which fully blocks the rewarding actions of heroin or morphine and thus makes their usage pointless. Unfortunately, naltrexone tends to lower mood, probably by blocking endogenous opioids or by acting at other receptors, and this lessens compliance. Two other problems exist with the use of naltrexone in addicts. The first is the risk of precipitating withdrawal when therapy is begun. The other is that if an addict wishes to reinstate the habit then it is possible to stop the antagonist, have a few shots, and restart the naltrexone again before going back to the clinic.

Another interesting application of opioid antagonists in preventing abuse is in combination with agonist analgesics in an attempt to prevent or reduce illicit use (diversion). Thus pentazocine/naloxone and buprenorphine/naloxone combinations are being tried as analgesics. The effects of the antagonist are insignificant when the combination is used orally for pain relief due to the poor bioavailability of the antagonist. However, if there is diversion and the drugs are injected by dependent addicts then the naloxone precipitates an aversive degree of withdrawal.

Some excitement was provoked a few years ago by the claim that a benzodiazepine receptor inverse agonist (Ro15–4513) behaved as a specific and selective antagonist of alcohol (Suzdak *et al*. 1986). On close inspection this claim was not fully substantiated although some efficacy was demonstrated, particularly in rats (see Lister and Nutt 1988). Unfortunately, any clinical potential of Ro15–4513 as an alcohol antagonist would have been excluded by its profound anxiogenic and proconvulsant actions. Nevertheless, the goal of finding a therapeutically useful alcohol antagonist is still one many espouse, especially if it could help decrease craving. Some recent animal work has raised again an old idea that opioid antagonists may decrease the acute rewarding actions of alcohol and so, if used repeatedly, could gradually produce an extinction of voluntary intake (Kornet *et al.* 1991). New clinical studies have offered support for this approach (O'Malley *et al.* 1993; Volpicelli *et al.* 1993).

Currently it is not established whether cannabis is acting as an agonist or antagonist at its receptor (see Marx 1990). If agonism is revealed then there would be a real potential for therapeutic interventions with antagonists. It is possible that the actions of LSD may be blocked by selective 5-HT antagonists (see Peroutka and Schmidt 1991), although there seems to be little interest in this line of approach. Perhaps the rising use of MDMA, which probably also acts, in part, through the 5-HT system will, if true dependence and craving becomes apparent, encourage a re-evaluation of this possibility. Finally, for completeness it should be noted that it is unlikely that antagonists will be a viable therapy for solvent abuse or caffeine use.

Finally, the role of availability in abuse potential should be appreciated. This is probably the most important factor in determining abuse of any drug and is one which, at least for the legally available agents, is under political control. It is well established that ease of access to alcohol determines the level of social damage caused by its abuse, and that usage is especially sensitive to pricing structure (see Godfrey this volume). Similarly, the high level of opioid addicts in the medical and pharmacy professions reflects easier availability of these drugs. Abuse of the benzodiazepines was significantly promoted by their being extensively prescribed coupled with the simultaneous decline in prescriptions for barbiturates. In general, the accessibility of street drugs has a large influence on the abuse potential, although stemming this supply may be more difficult than reducing usage by other strategies.

Is there a common process underlying abuse potential?

The quest for a unifying explanation for drug addiction has become something of a Holy Grail for preclinical researchers in this field. Several sorts of theories have emerged over the past few decades as our understanding of the pharmacology of addictive agents has blossomed. The discovery of endogenous opioids and their receptors in the 1970s led to suggestions that other addictive agents might also act through changes in this system. Thus theories in which alcohol contributed to the generation of endogenous opioid-like molecules came into vogue. A link with opioid systems was also demonstrated for some actions of the benzodiazepines. Recently, as mentioned above, the possibility that cocaine dependence might be related to opioid receptor function has been raised and this is now an area of active research.

In parallel with this line of approach has developed an understanding of the neuroanatomical substrate of drug abuse. The initiating observation was the dramatic demonstration that rats would self-administer electrical stimuli to certain brain regions. This led to the concept of a neural circuit that mediated reward or reinforcing behaviour linking parts of the limbic system, such as the nucleus accumbens and lateral hypothalamus. This was one of the greatest conceptual advances in neuroscience which has spawned many efforts to understand its neurochemical base. We now know that drugs such as the opioids, stimulants, and nicotine are rewarding if injected into these brain areas, and that animals will self-administer these drugs directly into these brain structures. It now appears that dopamine is an important, if not key, transmitter in the reward pathway, and there is a growing consensus that dopamine release in the nucleus accumbens is a necessary condition for any pleasurable activity including drug-induced reinforcement (Koob and Bloom 1988). The drugs which have most actions on dopamine (stimulants, opioids, alcohol, nicotine) tend to have the most abuse potential. In contrast, those with low abuse potential, such as the benzodiazepines and kappa-opioid agonists, do not increase dopamine release and may decrease it (Spanagel *et al.* 1990).

Further evidence for dopamine release being related to the processes of addiction is the finding that on chronic treatment there is an attenuation of the dopamine-releasing actions of the opioids but a sensitization to the effects of cocaine and amphetamine (Post and Kopanda 1976; and see Gawin 1991). Impressive as the accumbens–dopamine theory is it probably is not a sufficient explanation for addiction since drugs such as dopamine uptake blockers and monoamine oxidase inhibitors also increase dopamine availability in the brain but are not reinforcing (for example Colzi *et al.* 1990). Undoubtedly this field is one which will continue to develop, especially with the powerful new techniques of brain dialysis and *in situ* hybridization, to allow more precise analysis of the temporal and localization of the neurochemical circuits involved.

CONCLUSIONS

Pharmacology and its application to neuroscience continues to make a major impact on the understanding of addiction. These insights have changed our conceptualization of the nature of the addictive process and have produced a number of testable theories of the causes of tolerance and withdrawal. Moreover, applied pharmacology may lead to new or improved methods of treatment. Future efforts should be directed towards discovering the neurochemical mechanisms of craving (for example Benkelfat *et al.* 1991); this will require a concerted and integrated approach from both clinical and preclinical researchers.

ACKNOWLEDGEMENT

I thank Drs John Lewis and Bruce Holman for their very helpful comments.

REFERENCES

Aghajanian, G. K. (1978). Tolerance of locus coeruleus neurons to morphine and suppression of withdrawal response by clonidine. *Nature*, **276**, 186–8.

Benkelfat, C., Murphy, D. L., Hill, J. L., George, T. D., Nutt, D. J., and Linnoila, M. (1991). Ethanol-like properties of the serotonergic partial agonist *m*-chlorophenylpiperazine in chronic alcoholic patients. *Archives of General Psychiatry*, **48**, 383.

Colzi, A., d'Agostini, F., Kettler, R., Borroni, E., and Da Prada, M. (1990). Effect of selective and reversible MAO inhibitors on dopamine outflow in rat striatum: a microdialysis study. *Journal of Neural Transmitters* (Suppl.), **32**, 79–84.

Gallager, D. W., Heninger, K., and Heninger, G. (1986). Periodic benzodiazepine antagonist administration prevents benzodiazepine withdrawal symptoms in primates. *European Journal of Pharmacology*, **132**, 31–8.

Gawin, F. H. (1991). Cocaine addiction: psychology and neurophysiology. *Science*, 1580–6.

Glue, P. and Nutt, D. J. (1990). Overexcitement and disinhibition: dynamic neurotransmitter interactions in alcohol withdrawal. *British Journal of Psychiatry*, **157**, 491–9.

Goodman, A., Gilman, L. S., Rall, T. W., and Murad, F. (1985). *Goodman and Gilman's The pharmacological basis of therapeutics*. Macmillan Publishing Company, New York.

Griffiths, R. R., Bigelow, G. E., Liebsin, I., and Kaliszak, J. E. (1980). Drug reference in humans: double-blind choice comparison of pentobarbital, diazepam, and placebo. *Journal of Pharmacology and Experimental Therapeutics*, **215**, 649–61.

Griffiths, R. R., McLeod, D. R., Bigelow, G. E., Liebson, I., and Roache, J. D. (1984). Relative abuse liability of diazepam and oxazepam; behavioural and subjective dose effects. *Psychopharmacology*, **84**, 147–54.

Haigh, J. R. M. and Feely, M. (1988). Tolerance to the anticonvulsant effect of benzodiazepines. *Trends in Pharmacological Science*, **9**, 361–6.

Hernandez, T. D., Heninger, C., Wilson, M. A., and Gallager, D. W. (1989). Relationship of agonist efficacy to changes in GABA sensitivity and anticonvulsant tolerance following chronic benzodiazepine ligand exposure. *European Journal of Pharmacology*, **170**, 145–55.

Jasinski, D. A., Martin, W. R., and Haertzen, C. A. (1967). The human pharmacology and abuse potential of *N*-allylnoroxymorphone (Naloxone). *Journal of Pharmacology and Experimental Therapeutics*, **157**, 420–6.

Jasinski, D. R., Pevnick, J. S., and Griffith, J. D. (1978). Human pharmacology and abuse potential of the analgesic buprenorphine. *Archives of General Psychiatry*, **35**, 501–16.

Kennedy, C. and Henderson, G. (1991). μ-Opioid receptor inhibition of calcium current: development of homologous tolerance in single SH-SY5Y cells after chronic exposure to morphine *in vitro*. *Molecular Pharmacology*, **40**, 1000–5.

Koob, G. F. and Bloom, F. E. (1988). Cellular and molecular mechanisms of drug dependence. *Science*, **242**, 715–23.

Kornet, M., Goosen, C., and Van Ree, J. M. (1991). Effect of naltrexone on alcohol consumption during chronic alcohol drinking and after a period of imposed abstinence in free-choice drinking rhesus monkeys. *Psychopharmacology (Berlin)*, **104** (3), 367–76.

Kosten, T. R., Kleber, H. D., and Morgan, C. (1989). Treatment of cocaine abuse with buprenorphine *Biological Psychiatry*, **26**, 637–9.

Krystal, J. H., Walker, S. W., and Heninger, G. R. (1989). Intermittent naloxone administration decreases physical dependence on methadone in rhesus monkeys. *European Journal of Pharmacology*, **160**, 331–8.

Lister, R. G. and Nutt, D. J. (1988). Alcohol antagonists—the continuing quest. *Alcohol Clinical Experimental Research*, **12**, 566–9.

Marx, J. (1990). Marijuana receptor gene cloned. *Science*, **249**, 624–6.

Mello, N. K., Mendelson, J. H., Bree, M. P., and Lukas, S. E. (1989). Buprenorphine suppresses cocaine self-administration by rhesus monkeys. *Science*, **245**, 859–62.

Moreau, J. L., Jenck, F., Pieri, L., Schoch, P., Martin, J. R., and Haefely, W. E. (1990). Physical dependence induced in DBA/2J mice by benzodiazepine receptor full agonists, but not by the partial agonist Ro 16–6028. *European Journal of Pharmacology*, **190**, 269–73.

Nutt, D. J. (1990*a*). In: *Current aspects of the neurosciences* (ed. N. N. Osborne), pp. 259–93. Macmillan Press, London.

Nutt, D. J. (1990*b*). In: *Clinical aspects of panic disorder* (ed. J. C. Ballenger), pp. 281–96. Wiley-Liss, New York.

Nutt, D. J. and Costello, M. (1988). Rapid induction of lorazepam dependence and its reversal with flumazenil. *Life Science*, **43**, 1045–53.

Nutt, D. J. and Glue, P. (1986). Monoamines and alcohol. *British Journal of Addiction*, **81**, 327–38.

Nutt, D. J., Glue, P., Molyneux, S., and Clark, E. (1988). Alpha-2-adrenoceptor activity in alcohol withdrawal: a pilot study of the effects of i.v. clonidine in alcoholics and normals. *Alcohol Clinical Experimental Research*, **12**, 14–18.

O'Malley, S. S., Jaffe, A. J., Chang, G. Scholtenfeld, R. S., Meyer, R. E., and Rounsaville, B. (1993). Naltrexone and coping skills therapy for alcohol dependence: a controlled study. *Archives of General Psychiatry*, **49**, 881–7.

Peroutka, S. J. and Schmidt, A. W. (1991). In *5-Hydroxytryptamine in psychiatry —a spectrum of ideas* (ed. M. Sandler, A. Coppen, and S. Harnett). Oxford University Press, Oxford.

Post, R. M. and Kopanda, R. T. (1976). Cocaine, kindling and psychosis. *American Journal of Psychotherapy*, **133**, 627–34.

Siegel, S. (1976). Morphine analgesic tolerance: its situation specificity supports a Pavlovian conditioning model. *Science*, **193**, 323–5.

Siegel, S. (1984). Pavlovian conditioning and heroin overdose: reports by overdose victims. *Bulletin of the Psychonomic Society*, **22**, 428–30.

Silverstone, P. H. and Grahame-Smith, D. G. (1992). A review of the relationship between calcium channels and psychiatry. *Journal of Psychopharmacology*, **6**, 462–82.

Spanagel, R., Herz, A., and Shippenberg, T. S. (1990). The effects of opioid peptides on dopamine release in the nucleus accumbens: an *in vivo* microdialysis study. *Journal of Neurochemistry*, **55**, 1743–50.

Strain, E. C., Preston, K. L., Liebson, I. A., and Bigelow, G. E. (1992). The acute effects of buprenorphine, hydromorphone, and naloxone in methadone-maintained volunteers. *Journal of Pharmacology and Experimental Therapeutics*, **261**, 985–93.

Suzdak, P. D., Glowa, J. R., Crawley, J. N., Schwartz, R. D., Skolnick, P., and Paul, S. M. (1986). A selective imidazobenzodiazepine antagonist of ethanol in the rat. *Science*, **234**, 1243–7.

Volpicelli, J. R., Alterman, A. I., Hayashida, M. and O'Brien, C. P. (1993). Naltrexone in the treatment of alcohol dependence. *Archives of General Psychiatry*, **49**, 876–80.

4

Can psychology make sense of change?

ROBIN DAVIDSON

INTRODUCTION

Much of psychology is an attempt to understand the genesis and maintenance of behaviour, affect, cognitions, and attitudes as well as the conditions which facilitate transition. However, despite George Kelly's (1955) definition of psychology as the study of personal change there have been remarkably few texts specifically examining the nature of change. In one of these Watzlawick *et al.* (1974) argue that movement must be seen against a backdrop of the processes which maintain behaviour. Why do people **not** change what are obviously destructive self-defeating behaviour patterns? Persistence and change cannot be considered separately, as all perception, thought, and behaviour is relative and understood by comparison and contrast. Differing emphasis is placed on change resulting from maturation, environmental conditions, and personal intention, but the core questions of each branch of the discipline of psychology address these issues of behavioural persistence and change.

Developmental psychology, for example, is the study of maturational, mental, and social changes throughout the life cycle. We can chart a child's transition from reasoning logically to thinking symbolically. There is now an understanding about the impact on later life of early deprivation of social attachment. It would seem, as Kohlberg (1984) suggests, that individuals pass through different and prescribed stages of moral development. Developmental psychology has also afforded insights into the intellectual and cognitive sequelae of the journey through adulthood to old age.

Social psychology demonstrates the powerful contextual processes which promote behavioural persistence and change. For example, our social roles are regulated by norms about how someone in that position should behave. Three seminal social psychology studies from the early 1970s illustrate the importance of social roles and their profound influence on behavioural change. The students of Haney *et al.* (1973) became 'prisoners' and 'guards'. Hospital staff saw Rosenhams (1973) eight volunteers as 'psychiatric patients' and Milgrams (1974) sample became vigorous 'teachers'. Although these studies now look dated, artificial, and simplified they are a continuing testament to the behavioural changes which role manipulation can induce. The early Solomon Asch (1965) studies on conformity have been followed by decades of research which more or less confirms that people will behave in a group very differently to the way they would on their own. Aranson (1988) summarizes the reasons for this which include group identification, the wish to be liked, the desire for personal gain, and the sometimes irrational acceptance of what others say and do. Recent studies demonstrate graphically the variables which contribute to significant behavioural and attitudinal change arising from membership of coercive groups such as religious cults. The book by Robert Cialdini (1988) on the weapons of social influence should be required reading for all who are in the business of facilitating change in others. Of particular interest to addiction workers are his observations on the processes of commitment and consistency. Once a choice or stand is made there are interpersonal pressures to behave consistently with that commitment. Cialdini summarises this work and lists a variety of elements which contribute to making commitment effective in constraining or modifying future behaviour. Public, written, incremental, effortful and internally motivated factors are those which would seem to strengthen commitment to change.

The central concern of personality theory and resultant psychotherapies is clearly that of behavioural persistence and change. Some years ago Milton Erikson (1974) noted that people generally do not seek psychotherapy for reasons of enlightenment about the unchangeable past but rather because of dissatisfaction with the present and a desire to better the future. More recently, Phares (1992) said much the same when he defined psychotherapy as psychological interventions which induce changes in a person's behaviour, thoughts, or feelings.

The above discussion illustrates the ubiquity of ideas about persistence and change in psychology. Rather than a broad discussion of these throughout psychology the primary focus of this chapter will be on those aspects which help us understand individual behavioural change and how such change is maintained over time. The sometimes oblique relationship between psychological theory and practice will also be examined. Psychotherapies based on analytical theories which explore personal growth, insight, and gradual awareness of unconscious conflicts through reconstruction of the personality are evaluated elsewhere.

One of the key issues is the move, particularly in clinical psychology, from the more deterministic view of change espoused by radical behaviourists towards a cognitive position which emphasizes volition and intention. Because of the central importance of this cognitive approach to persistence and change most of this chapter will be devoted to some of the contemporary cognitive themes within psychology and their influence in understanding processes of change within addiction. Consideration will also be given to phenomenological perspectives which have become increasingly influential in the field of addiction. However, in order to place these in context the first section is a brief discussion of the more traditional behavioural view of change.

A BEHAVIOURIST PERSPECTIVE

The radical behaviourist approach to therapeutic change is characterized more than anything by a putative commitment to the guiding principles of experimental research. Criticisms of the behaviourist position as lacking reflexivity, reductionist, mechanistic, and deterministic are well known. More succinct is Kelly's (1969) comment that a 'psychopath is a stimulus—response psychologist who takes it seriously'. On the other hand contemporary proponents of radical behaviourism, of whom Rescorla (1988) is arguably the most vociferous, say that there is a richness within conditioning models not envisioned within the reflex tradition. Conditioning is seen as learning arising from exposure to associations among environmental events and is the primary means whereby an individual represents the structure of his or her world. Wherever the truth lies there are a number of change strategies employed by addiction therapists which lend themselves to parsimonious explanation in the language of conditioning. Perhaps the most well known is cue exposure.

Cue exposure

Cue exposure is generally understood in terms of both classical and operant conditioning. Drug responses which can include withdrawal symptoms (Wikler 1965), agonistic effects (Stewart *et al.* 1984), antagonistic or compensatory effects (Siegel 1988), and opponent processes (Donovan and Chaney 1985) become associated with aspects of the internal or external environment. Environmental cues become conditioned stimuli which when presented in the absence of the unconditioned stimulus can potentially produce this variety of conditioned responses. After classical conditioning, instrumental learning is said to occur as the conditioned responses become discriminative stimuli, that is they become motivatory and modulate continued drug using behaviour. Cue exposure, should theoretically extinguish the conditioned response and so alter future behaviour. In their summary of 20 years of cue exposure research Drummond *et al.* (1990) conclude, rather disappointingly, that no study has unambiguously demonstrated its efficacy in promoting long term, good quality change in the behaviour of dependent drinkers. This is arguably due to the fact that no studies have taken full account of the range of conditions which are theoretically necessary to produce change in the drinkers operant responses. There should be greater emphasis on individual differences in cue reactivity and in the varying pattern of physiological responses to specific environmental cues. Only salient stimuli should be included if generalization of response is to occur in the individuals natural environment. For example, the prediction of conditioning models is that cue exposure conducted in a natural setting, without a therapist and with only the most individually salient cues employed would promote generalization. Foa and Kozak (1986) in their work with anxious patients noted that long-term habituation is enhanced when people are, for example, instructed to focus on the most salient aspects of the stimuli. It is also predicted that despite possible response desyncrony, within session habituation should maximize the possibility of longer term change. In practice this means individually tailored cues of varying duration with preset criteria for the termination of each session. Recent studies with opiate addicts (Powell *et al.* 1993) which have taken account of these variables have produced promising results, while the introduction of cognitive variables did not significantly improve the procedure.

Cue exposure is an example of a treatment for which conditioning models neatly predict the optimum conditions for change. Future exposure programmes, as Drummond *et al.* (1990) suggest, should be allied to basic non-clinical research, a point which is essentially the theme of this chapter.

Aversion conditioning

A second example of a treatment based explicitly on conditioning principles is emetic therapy or chemical aversion which is said to decrease the appetitive allure of alcohol and drugs (Wilson 1991). The history of this can be traced as far back as Rush (1789) who after administering rum containing a tartar emetic found that his patient 'could not bear the sight or smell of spirits for two years afterwards'. On the face of it this would seem to be an example of long-standing, good quality, behavioural change. It is clear from the work of Garcia (1989) and others that not all stimuli are equally as associable, or in Seligman's (1970) terms there is differential 'associative preparedness'. Aversion involving nausea is a well-established, adaptive, and efficient learning process, and the following discussion will focus on chemical rather than electrical aversion. Cannon *et al.* (1981) demonstrate the superiority of chemical aversion and Elkins (1991) rationalizes why theoretically it would be predicted to produce better results.

Despite numerous anecdotal reports there have been few well-controlled outcome studies which demonstrate the efficacy of emetic therapy in producing long term behavioural change. However, as with cue exposure the most interesting deficits are theoretical rather than methodological. For example, the temporal continuity between the conditioned and unconditioned stimuli is important. Some unsuccessful applications may be the result of alcohol introduction to the patient after the peak of nausea (Elkins 1991). The number and frequency of booster sessions is also critical. Those studies which have employed reasonable sound conditioning procedures demonstrate fairly good results, and most independent reviewers, for example, Nathan (1985) conclude that it can be a moderately effective change procedure for some drinkers. Arguably, however, there is only one outcome study which is theoretically and methodologically flawless (Cannon and Baker 1981). Here there was random assignment of subjects to aversive and non-aversive treatment conditions with optimal conditioned stimulus/ unconditioning stimulus intervals being employed. This study provides clear support for the use of chemical aversion as part of an alcohol treatment package.

Covert sensitization (verbal aversion) is often suggested as an alternative to drug-induced nausea, and Hester and Miller (1989) have helpfully outlined practical recommendations for the implementation of covert sensitization. While some studies have shown it to be no better than alternative interventions, for example Piorkowski and Mann (1975), others have demonstrated that clients who unambiguously experience conditioned nausea responses remain abstinent longer than those who do not (Elkins 1980). Covert sensitization offers the advantage of not requiring drug administration and so makes aversion therapy available to a wider range of clients.

Of course the criticism of aversive procedures is well founded. It can be inhumane and seen as pejorative (Wilson 1991). However, the importance of aversive procedures in the present context is that they are informed by conditioning theory and again the conditions for maximum change can be specified.

The change processes arising from cue exposure and aversion therapy have been at times re-interpreted in cognitive terms such as enhancement of self-efficacy and mastery. Eysenck (1987) would say, however, that cognitive change is simply a consequence of behaving in a different way and that the effects of cognitive and behavioural intervention are so confounded that it is impossible to make a judgement about their relative efficacy. In the general treatment literature, particularly on anxiety-based problems, many studies have found little difference in outcome when cognitive and purely behavioural approaches are compared (Marks 1987; Latimer and Sweet 1984). Indeed in their review Parloff *et al.* (1986) found that for some problem drinkers aversion therapy was consistently better than more cognitively based interventions at one year follow-up. Furthermore, the work of Levey and Martin (1987) indicates that contingency awareness does not necessarily enhance the strength of association. In a slightly different context Heather and Stallard (1989) argue that contemporary cognitive models tend to underestimate the importance of classically conditioned craving in the relapse process. If conditioning formulations are systematically operationalized, if the constructs are linked together, and if a set of conditions is predicted which maximize change, it seems to add little to our understanding of **specific and focused** conditioning based strategies, such as cue exposure and aversion training, to invoke less systematic cognitive explanations. Increasingly however, therapists are using less focused interventions which cannot easily be understood in stimulus response terms. The person who is changing must have acquired **knowledge** about the association between stimuli rather than just having learned to behave in a different way. The next section examines some cognitive components of change.

A COGNITIVE PERSPECTIVE

Background

Many learning theorists, for example Papini and Bitterman (1990) have rejected even Rescorla's (1988) sophisticated rationalization of conditioning theory and would argue that activities such as information seeking, preconceptions, attribution, and expectancy must necessitate a more cognitive view of learning and motivation. Apart from the general criticisms of the behavioural perspective noted above, there have been many findings in learning experiments over the years which have had to call on increasingly convoluted and unconvincing behavioural explanations. Latent learning, which is not expressed immediately and occurs without reinforcement, is one such area of study. When the reinforcer is eventually introduced it must act merely as a motivator to access already existing knowledge. Indeed it was latent learning experiments which led the doyen of cognitive psychologists, Tolman (1948), to talk in terms of cognitive maps. Neither can observational and insight learning be satisfactorily explained in stimulus–response terms as they must take account of knowledge about responses and their consequences.

Because of these and other anomalies much of contemporary psychology is grounded on cognitive foundations. Cognitive psychology is an attempt to describe and explain how new knowledge is acquired, internally represented, and influences future behaviour. The emphasis is on mental processes which intervene between stimulus and response. Mahoney (1988) defines cognitive psychology

as a family of theories which share the assertion that human knowledge and experience entail the proactive participation of the individual.

It is probably fair to say that the majority of pure and applied psychologists studying areas as diverse as perception, reasoning, memory language, and motivation would see themselves as cognitively orientated.

Experimental cognitive psychology is generally considered to include the investigation of perception and memory. The latter, for example, is now seen as a processor in which information is not passively recorded but actively altered and organized thus building up increasingly complex cognitive schemas (Wade and Tavris 1993). The branch of cognitive psychology which is most relevant to the present discussion is what Brewin (1988) describes as 'social cognition'. This is essentially the study of how information about oneself and others is registered and processed. Its roots lie in the work of social psychologists such as Lewin (1947) and Heider (1958), and it is probably not an exaggeration to say that in the past two decades clinical psychology, at least in the United Kingdom and North America, has become almost exclusively 'social cognition' orientated.

Theory and practice

There are a considerable number of theories and therapies which are broadly cognitive in nature. In his review Dobson (1988) counted over 20 different types of cognitive therapy. Winter (1992) points out that there often appears to be little connection between cognitive therapy and cognitive psychology. Brewin (1989) also notes that cognitive therapy systems are often at best only tenuously based on experimental research and theorizing in cognitive and social psychology, while Smith (1982) warns against indiscriminate selection of bits and pieces from diverse sources which results in a hodge podge of inconsistent concepts and techniques.

These criticisms may be a little overstated as influential cognitive therapy systems such as those of Beck (1976) and Ellis (1962) do, to some extent, draw on general psychology findings from the reasoning, problem solving, and information processing. Nevertheless, the prevailing criticism that diverse cognitive approaches to understanding persistence and change have the potential for theoretical chaos has prompted Phares (1992) to call for a systematic theoretical position that will incorporate all cognitive change strategies and will help the therapist decide under what conditions to employ one technique rather than another. This search for an integrating framework is the theme of Brewin's (1989) paper on cognitive change processes. Here he emphasizes the importance of automatic and controlled information processing and distinguishes between knowledge which is verbally accessible and that which can only be gained by exposure to situational cues. Brewin also identifies a number of mechanisms of cognitive change which should be specified before designing a cognitive therapy intervention. His integrated model of change draws on converging lines of evidence and represents an attempt to relate cognitive behavioural therapy to experimental research in cognitive and social psychology.

A related issue is the internal theoretical rigour of various social cognition approaches to treatment and change. For example, Rotters (1975) work is quite systematic, while Bandura's (1977) social learning theory has been criticized as consisting of a loose collection of processes and concepts, highly descriptive and lacking specification of exactly how it works (Phares 1992). Given this criticism it is slightly worrying that in the mid 1980s social learning theory was hailed by some as a Kuhnian paradigm shift in our conceptualization of addiction. The term social learning theory, although first coined by Dollard and Miller (1950), generally refers to the work of Bandura and Rotter. This is only part of the array of ideas which constitute social cognition.

At the risk of over simplification cognitive approaches to the understanding of behavioural persistence and change can be classified under a number of headings. The **expectancy value** framework could include, for example, Bandura's social learning theory, Rotter's work on locus of control in which he examined generalized expectancies for internal or external control of reinforcement, the health belief model of Becker and Maiman (1975) and Seligman's (1975) original formulation of learned helplessness. The **explanation attribution** framework could include motivational models such as those of Weiner (1985), Feather (1982), and Davies (1992) which link causal attribution to motivational processes of intensity, directionality, and persistence of behaviour. Later formulations of learned helplessness are also couched in attributional terms (Abramson *et al*. 1978). While helplessness may be an efficacy expectation following an experience of uncontrollability, more important is a person's understanding of **why** the uncontrollable experience occurred. Beck's cognitive behaviour therapy which challenges depressogenic assumptions is also attributional in emphasis. A **reasoned action** framework refers to those approaches which posit that behaviour change is preceded by intention. This could, I suppose, include the Janis and Mann (1977) view of decision making being based on a kind of mental balance sheet, D'Zurilla and Goldfried's (1971) problem solving and the self-regulation approach of Meichenbaum (1977) and others.

In order to structure this discussion cognitive approaches to change will be summarized under these, albeit fairly arbitrary, headings. Many authors, for example Orford (1985) and Davidson (1991), have noted that treatment processes are not necessarily distinct from the naturally occurring change strategies employed by so-called self changers. These, mainly cognitive strategies are not qualitatively distinct from those described in formal therapeutic systems. While much of this chapter focuses on strategies drawn from the treatment literature it should be remembered that they are only part of the wider picture of change and that many people who deal with a problem do so without recourse to formal treatment (Tuchfeld 1976; Saunders and Kershaw 1979).

Expectancy value framework

As noted above it is difficult to categorize cognitive treatment approaches as most therapy systems use a cocktail of techniques. These usually include verbal persuasion, attempts to alter self-appraisal, and the attenuation of habitual thought patterns and behaviour. However, theories which emphasize expectancy have been particularly influential in the development of change processes with addictions.

The relapse prevention model of Marlatt and Gordon (1985) is a combination of strategies aimed at promoting and maintaining change. They include enhancing awareness of the vagaries of change, coping skills training, advice on a balanced life-style, and the development of more constructive attributions about abstinence violation. Their emphasis is quite explicitly, however, on the promotion of change in efficacy and outcome expectations. The criticism of their model of relapse prevention by Edwards (1987) as an 'artificial segmentation of the interacting and fluctuating process of change' has been acknowledged by Marlatt and Gordon (1989) in their later description of relapse as part of the process of behaviour change. Like Prochaska and Di Clemente (1983) they argue that the habit change process is a series of interlocking stages and that a relapse prevention approach can be applied at any time as either an intervention or prevention strategy. It is said to extend beyond the immediate need to intervene at a particular point in the change process and will ultimately enrich quality of life as a correlate of habit change.

The other influential relapse prevention model is that of Annis and Davis (1989) who are quite clear that Bandura's self-efficacy theory is the framework which has specifically guided their strategies for initiation and enhancement of permanent change. Accordingly, rather than discuss these relapse prevention models it is more apposite to offer a brief critique of Bandura's theory.

Bandura (1977) argues that self-efficacy is an attempt to provide a unified account of change resulting from various psychological therapies, the most successful of which are those which are said to maximize efficacy beliefs. An efficacy expectation is one's view that he or she can perform a task successfully, while an outcome expectation is the belief that a given behaviour **will produce** a particular outcome. Efficacy beliefs are said to develop in four ways. First is a result of past experience of success and failure, second is vicarious learning through the observation of others in similar situations, third is verbal persuasion, and the fourth arises from an individual's experience of emotional arousal. This final pathway is based on the observation that perceived anxiety can reduce an individual's expectation of performing a task successfully. The converse of this is that reduced fear arousal has been shown to increase self-efficacy in phobic individuals. Bandura (1982) cites evidence from various sources in support of his assertion that successful behavioural change is more than just differential exposure to the problem situation and that there is a correlation between strength of efficacy belief and successful behavioural change, at least in specific if not more diffuse and complex target behaviours.

In his excellent summary of the evidence for the self-efficacy theory, Brewin (1988) concludes that its predictive power is maximized when the criteria for successful performance are unambiguous and when the necessary behaviour is under deliberate conscious control. In other words no amount of efficacy belief that one can play bass guitar in a rock band will help if the individual is tone deaf. So people may make valid efficacy judgements under certain limited conditions but at the end of the day these may be little more than **statements of intention**. Common sense tells us that the person who says he is going to perform a task will probably be able to do it. This implies that there is no causal relationship between efficacy belief as such and subsequent behaviour. The charge that efficacy judgements are nothing more than statements of intention is difficult to refute on current evidence although the success of efficacy judgements in predicting longer term behavioural change would go some way to militating against a simple intention explanation.

A final issue is the idea that efficacy beliefs are driven by what Bandura calls 'self referent thoughts'. They are based on conscious thought processes and so limited by an individual's lack of access to learned associations which are outside his or her conscious awareness. This is in contrast to conditioning models which would predict, for example, that conditioned consummatory aversion can occur without the individual being aware of what caused the aversion (Logue 1985).

Explanation attribution framework

While the expectancy perspective is squarely based on findings from experimental psychology, the development of attribution theory can be traced to the ideas of social psychologists such as Heider (1958). In one sense attributions can be seen as reciprocally related to expectations. Attribution theorists assume that individuals deliberately attempt to explain events in order to maximize future control (Cheng and Nowik 1990). Particular types of explanation are said to optimize a person's ability to alter their behaviour in the face of adverse circumstances. Causal beliefs are essentially hypotheses about cause/effect relationships which are formed from a constellation of previous experiences and brought to bear on one's behavioural repertoire when facing a current complex or difficult situation.

Different theorists describe attribution as varying across a number of dimensions. For example, **situational attribution** implies that the individual accords causal status to something in the environment, while **dispositional attribution** is concerned with intrapersonal traits. If the subjects in Stanley Milgram's experiments thought of themselves as sadists this would be a dispositional explanation. If however, as is more likely, they viewed themselves as having been manipulated by an unscrupulous experimenter they would be applying a situational explanation. In general when explaining one's own behaviour most people employ attributions favourable to themselves. This so-called self-serving bias has been discussed by many authors, for example Markus and Kitayama (1991). Like stereotyping, attributions are heuristics which people use to organize information about the world which might otherwise be overwhelming.

Weiner's (1986) motivational model posits that attributional hypotheses differ on three main dimensions, namely internality/externality, stability/instability, and controllability/uncontrollability. The dimensions of attribution of *Abramson et al.* (1978) are arguably the most well known and not dissimilar to those of *Weiner*. **Stable** attributions are those in which the cause is seen as a result of something relatively permanent and unchanging, **global** attributions are those in which the cause is perceived to influence many situations, and **internal** attribution ascribes cause to personal rather than external variables. Traditionally attribution theorists have tended to investigate mood states and health-related behaviour, although the principles of attribution have also been applied to our understanding of addictive behaviour (Eiser 1983; Davies 1992).

Davies (1992) has challenged what he calls the 'myth' of addiction by specifically applying attributional principles to drug use. He emphasizes volition rather than compulsion, rejecting the idea of the 'helpless addict'. He also makes the familiar point that bias can be introduced to personal explanations of behaviour as a result of individual differences in motives, contexts, and intentions. In assessing the validity of any attributions the functional significance for the individual must be taken into account. Dissonance, for example, may be reduced if the drug user can explain his behaviour in terms of personal addiction defined as an interaction between stable and internal attributions. In other words, drug using behaviour is seen as a result of personal and enduring characteristics thus reducing the possibility of future change. This personal attributional system tends to place excessive drug use beyond volition and absolves the individual of responsibility. Addiction is not, Davies argues, a 'thing which happens to people but a functional set of cognitions surrounding the activity of taking drugs'. He appeals for a change in the constellation of attributions which is generally applied to explain excessive drug use. Only then can people be imbued with the personal power to promote a sense of control and set in place the conditions for altering problematic behaviour.

Fosterling (1985) reviewed the literature on attribution retraining. Despite theoretical prediction there has been little good experimental demonstration of reframed attributions specifically promoting change in future drug using behaviour.

There is a danger here in rejecting addiction as a myth and substituting it with a general explanation of drug use in terms of attribution. Edwards (1993) reminds us that addiction is multifactorial and points out the pitfalls of touting all encompassing explanations in the language of a single discipline or theory. Furthermore, while for some people a personal theory of addiction may not make sense of their own experience, for others it surely does. For this latter group it is the belief that they **are** addicts which inspires faith and promotes change (Keene and Raynor 1993).

Reasoned action framework

Change can be seen in terms of reasoned decision making. Janis and Mann (1977) in their psychological analysis of conflict, choice, and commitment suggested that motivation for change arises when losses occurring from a behaviour exceed the gains, thus prompting the individual to seek out new solutions. This is underpinned by the idea that behavioural change and persistence is characterized by conflict or in behavioural terms, approach/avoidance. Orford (1985) draws on the work of Janis and Mann as part of his general account of the psychology of excessive appetites in which he argues that reasoned action arising from conflict or dissonance is the central motivating component of the change process.

Reasoned action towards change can also be promoted by problem solving. This consists of a number of processes including enhancing self-awareness, reducing personal chaos, and working towards constructive solutions. The so-called 'problem solving' strategies outlined in the chapters on treatment at the end of most addiction texts are loosely based on the general psychology principles of thought, creativity, and language. D'Zurilla and Goldfried's (1971) work on the five constituent stages of problem solving is the framework most commonly used in the treatment of self-perceived problematic behaviour. The approach is based on the idea that reasoning is a purposeful mental activity which involves operating on information to reach conclusions. Wessells (1982) demonstrated four steps in the same process. Once the problem is recognized one clearly defines the problem, devises a strategy, executes the strategy, and then evaluates progress towards the goal. He goes on to draw the distinction between algorithms and heuristics. The former is problem solving by rules and prescribed strategies, while the latter is a course of action which may be right but does not guarantee an optimal solution. It could be speculated that treatment-induced change may be more akin to an algorithm, a sort of cook book approach to problem solving, while self-changers make more use of heuristic strategies.

Experimental psychologists have identified a number of barriers to problem solving including rigid mental set and functional fixedness, and Beck (1976) has drawn on this work in his description of depressogenic thoughts and assumptions.

A related set of strategies employed to facilitate change are those which enhance self-regulation. Kanfer (1986) defines this as 'planful action designed to change the course of one's behaviour'. Here the individual, whether through therapy or personal inductive reasoning, develops a set of strategies which constitute a self-regulatory system. Meichenbaum (1977) developed what he called stress inoculation training in which he emphasized the importance of internal dialogue. Kirschenbaum (1987) also argues that we must pay systematic attention to self-monitoring, self-evaluation, and self-reinforcement.

Recently Diaz and Fruhauf (1991) have presented a developmental model of self-regulation which is of interest to workers in addiction. Like Brewin (1989) this draws a distinction between executive and automatic self-regulation with the latter referring primarily to arousal and attentional systems. They also see **self-control** as a rigid response system to externally determined directives, while **self-regulation** is more about achieving goals which are self-determined. In other words, the child develops from internalizing care giver's directions (self-control) to actually taking on the care giver's role (self-regulation). There are individual differences in the nature of this transition in that environments which are either too permissive or too controlling tend to stunt the development of self-regulation. The work of the developmental psychologist, Wertsch (1984), graphically illustrates these individual differences in a child's sense of mastery or competence. Adult vulnerability in self-regulatory function can be seen as, at least in part, a result of less than optional development (Block *et al*. 1988).

Strategies such as problem solving and enhancement of self-regulation are based on the view that under the right circumstances an individual can reasonably act in his or her own best interest. Again emphasis is on awareness and volition which allows for the individual to make choices and decisions.

THE PHENOMENOLOGICAL PERSPECTIVE

Background

The phenomenological approach to individual change, popularized particularly by Rogers (1951), can be traced to the European existentialism. This approach was at one time regarded as the 'third force' in psychology made up of people who were dissatisfied with the excesses of psychoanalysis and the reductionism of the behaviourist tradition. Man is basically seen as having choice and as intentional. Stress is placed in the individual's inner and present experience with the subjective 'self' being the core component of personal change and development. The American phenomenologists were rather more optimistic than the European existentialists. Rogers, for example saw the potential for growth in everyone and change as a process of self-actualization. His is the most complete, clearly articulated and systematic phenomenological theory. It is presented in a proposition form although some of the constructs are vague and difficult to operationalize. Essentially behaviour is seen as a goal-directed activity for the enhancement of the 'self'. More recently client centred therapists (Markus and Worf 1987) have, like cognitive psychologists, discussed self-schemas which are gradually built up through experience to help process self-regulated and self-congruent information. There is also the well-known emphasis on a democratic relationship between client and helper, with therapist variables such as accurate empathy, unconditional positive regard, and congruence being regarded as important catalysts of-change. There are, however, surprisingly few well-controlled outcome studies specifically examining the importance of these variables in producing good quality change. Lambert *et al*. (1978) and Lafferty *et al*. (1989) did find a small, but nevertheless significant, relationship between therapist variables and therapeutic effectiveness. Truax and Mitchell (1971), Miller and Baca (1983), and others have more specifically demonstrated the importance of accurate empathy in promoting resolution and change. On the other hand Rachman and Wilson (1980) would argue that there is a tendency to overemphasize the importance of therapist variables at the expense of treatment strategies and the psychology of individual differences.

Motivational interviewing

Motivational interviewing has been described as the most important and influential therapeutic development within the field of addiction over the last decade (Stockwell 1992). Motivational interviewing is, however, something of a misnomer as it has little to do with traditional or indeed contemporary cognitive theories of motivation. It seems rather to be an example of a phenomenological, humanistic approach to change, directly adapting the psychology of self-actualization to personal change among problem drug and alcohol users. Motivational interviewing eschews the traditional confrontational approach and apparent 'lack of motivation' is seen as a product of this style of therapist/client dialogue rather than an intrapersonal characteristic. Motivational interviewers define motivation simply as the probability that a person will enter into, continue, and adhere to a specific change strategy. The individual decides that change is in his or her best interest and the role of the therapist is to facilitate this decision through clarification, advice, accurate feedback, and empathy. There is a strong emphasis on role ambivalence in the decisional balance. Essentially, responsibility for decision making and change rests with the client, while the therapist sets the optimum conditions for change. The client begins to present his or her own arguments for change rather than being coerced by a directive therapist. Miller and Rollnick (1991) make a point of contrasting this and the Rogerian approach by in a sense caricaturing the neo-Rogerian position. They say, for example, that empathic reflection is invariably and non-contingently employed in client-centred counselling but used only selectively in motivational interviewing. The non-directive counsellor is said to avoid giving advice while the motivational interviewer will not be afraid to proffer advice when appropriate and will actively attempt to create discomfort and discrepancy rather than passively follow the client.

Winter (1992) however, notes that most post-Rogerian client-centred approaches are much more active and task-orientated than was originally the case. The therapist is less non-directional and acts as a 'surrogate information processor' which in turn facilitates the client to elaborate and re-organize his or her construction. Takens (1987) also comments that contemporary client-centred therapists are less benign and more focused during therapy. This would seem to imply that any distinction between motivational interviewing and client-centred counselling is little more than semantic, which is no bad thing. Motivational interviewing can be regarded as a good example of a therapeutic system specifically tailored to individual change in addictive behaviour but squarely based on psychological theory. There are now a number of studies appearing, for example Saunders and Allsop (1991), which demonstrate the power of motivational interviewing to enhance the resolution of alcohol and drug users.

The behavioural, cognitive, and phenomenological approaches presented above represent only a sample of frameworks used to generate the numerous contemporary psychotherapeutic strategies, although they are perhaps the most relevant to our current thinking in addiction. There is a history in psychology of attempted synthesis or the pulling together of recurring themes and processes of change. The next section reviews some of this work.

COMMON THEMES

Psychotherapy in its broadest sense has been defined by Meltzoff and Kornreich (1970) as

informed and planful application of techniques derived from established psychological principles ... with the intention of assisting individuals to modify such personal characteristics as feelings, values, attitudes and behaviour.

The work of Dollard and Miller (1950), Lazurus (1975), and Wachtel (1977) are important milestones in the literature on commonalties between psychoanalytic and behavioural approaches to change. Goldfried and Safran (1986) note that psychotherapy of the 1980s was characterized by integration and eclecticism, although this movement towards identification of common themes is not without its critics. Smail (1983) reminds us that psychotherapists are split into a variety of different schools with what he regards as fundamentally different and often mutually exclusive ideas. Hildebrand (1983) argues that the so-called therapeutic shopping basket leads to theoretical weakness, *ad hoc* hypotheses, and to assertion rather than careful evaluation. Arguably English and English (1958) articulated the compromise position when they commended integration as an orderly combination of compatible features from diverse sources. On the other hand, they dismiss unsystematic and uncritical combination as 'syncretism'.

One of the earliest papers searching for common change themes across the psychotherapies was that of Bibring (1952) who describes the basic concepts which can be applicable to all types of psychotherapy. He draws a distinction between technical factors and curative application of principles. The former are classified as suggestive, abreactive, manipulative, classificatory, and interpretive. He goes on to outline four simple types of curative processes:

(1) the production of material;

(2) the utilization of this material;

(3) the assimilation by the patient of the results of such utilization.

(4) the process of re-orientation and re-adjustment.

More recently authors such as Goldfried (1980) and Bergen (1980) have resumed the search for integrative models, and Goldfried and Robins (1982) suggest that rapprochement starts with the identification of common processes of change. Prochaska (1979) isolated some of the core processes common to a variety of psychotherapeutic systems which he said can be applied either experimentally or environmentally. Each process is basically a category of treatment activities which have something in common. His category of 'consciousness raising' can illustrate this (Davidson 1991). Examples within this cluster of activities could include the didactic approach of the educationalist, the confrontation of the rational emotive therapist, the video feedback of the behaviourist, or the interpretations of the analyst. This work was taken further by Prochaska and Di Clemente (1983) in a factor analytic study which isolated the ten independent processes of change summarized in Table 4.1. Like 'consciousness raising' most of these are self-explanatory, but as Ryle (1984) suggests individual therapy systems will emphasize only a few of the processes. 'Self'- and 'social'-liberation indicate an increased capacity for an individual to choose options. Counter conditioning and stimulus control refer to reduction in the strength of conditioned stimuli which would increase the probability of the erstwhile

TABLE 4.1 *The catalysts of change*

---

1. Consciousness raising
2. Self-re-evaluation
3. Environmental re-evaluation
4. Self-liberation
5. Social liberation
6. Counter-conditioning
7. Stimulus control
8. Contingency management
9. Dramatic relief
10. Helping relationships

---

problem responses reoccurring. Contingency management describes the altering of contingencies between response and reinforcement. Dramatic relief is similar to Belring's abreactive factor and is described as a rather sudden cathartic change evoked by observing or experiencing emotional events. Finally the helping relationship covers all of the issues inherent in the client/helper interaction which facilitate change. Despite the comments of Rachman and Wilson (1980) noted above, this category may be the most important of all. It is the view of this author that an emphasis on technique rather than the personal relationship between client and helper will ultimately detract from our full understanding of the processes of change.

THE STAGES OF CHANGE

The idea that stages in the process of change can be identified and operationalized straddles various branches of psychology. While some models address change in systems and others personal change, most include some variation on the core stages of resistance, re-adaption, and consolidation. Despite different frames of reference it is the similarities rather that the differences which are striking. Some examples will help highlight this.

There is a substantial literature on the nature of organizational change, and indeed nearly half a century ago Lewin (1947) presented his model of institutionalization which consisted of three phases in the change process. **Unfreezing** involves making the need for change apparent so that it can be accepted by the individual, group, or organization. **Moving** is the replacement of old values, attitudes and behaviours with new ones, while **refreezing** involves locking in the new behaviours. In their excellent and empirically supported model of workplace change based on the Lewin original, Buller *et al.* (1985) identify variables which contribute to persistence and change at each of the three stages.

At an individual level social psychologists have identified stages in attitudinal change. Cross (1971) looked at the development of racial identity among a cohort of black Americans. In what was termed the Negro to Black conversion experience, they charted the process of change from an insecure to a secure racial identity. The four stages of this process, later to be validated in a factor analytic study (Ponterotto and Wise 1987), were described as pre-encounter, immersion, emmersion, and internalization. This study has been discussed in more detail elsewhere, (Davidson 1991).

Psychotherapists have long been interested in the process of therapeutically-induced change. Pentony (1981) commented that most change through therapy involves an initial destructuring when resistance is examined and challenged, an intermediate stage of conversion culminating in the final stage of restructuring. George Kelly's (1955) constructionist view of change is one of the most clearly enunciated and it is his work which is the basis of many contemporary ideas on the processes and stages of personal change. Kelly was less concerned with the determinants of an individual's personality but rather emphasized the nature of change, its functional significance for the individual, and the conditions under which it occurs. Personal construct theorists would say that all of our present interpretations are subject to revision or replacement. Construing is an ongoing process in which we constantly revise our view of the world and consequently our behaviour. The core construct system is central to a person's identity and maintenance of a sense of 'self'. When this is challenged and the individual is expected to behave in an entirely new way 'threat' or 'anxiety' is experienced. Kelly describes the latter as a recognition that events with which we are confronted lie outside the range of convenience of our construct system. Anxiety is, therefore, a sign that revision is necessary. McCoy (1981) has also defined guilt and fear in personal construct terms and these too can at times be precursors of change. These are the conditions under which revision of behaviour can begin to occur. Kelly (1970) described the process of transition after this initial challenge as the Circumspection, Pre-emption, Control (CPC) cycle.

Once the conditions of change are in place, in the circumspection stage the various options are reviewed. During the next stage the person is said to construe pre-emptively or in other words focus on a particular issue at a time. Winter (1992) defines a pre-emptive construct as one which when applied to an event does not allow the application of any other construct. The control phase is a time when choices are made. Kelly (1970) also describes the Experience cycle, which is probably the

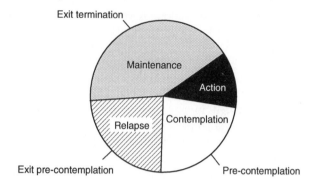

FIG. 4.1 Stages of individual change (after Prochaska and Di Clemente 1984).

core of personal construct theory, and describes rather longer term, more general change than the CPC cycle. At the risk of simplification its first stage is said to be Anticipation when a prediction is made. In the Pre-encounter phase the individual acts on this prediction, and then personal assessment is said to take place in the Confirmation or Disconfirmation phase. Finally in the Constructive revision stage the person reconstrues following evaluation of the experiences.

The notions of transitional stages and dispositional states have had some considerable influence on current thinking in addiction. Tuchfeld (1976) outlined a two-stage model of change after his detailed interviews with over 50 former problem drinkers. Kanfer and Grimm (1980) identified a number of critical transition points where individuals define themselves as in need of change and then attempt to act on this re-definition.

Perhaps the most well-known stage of change model within addictions is that of Prochaska and Di Clemente (1984). This is summarized in Fig. 4.1. The model was originally developed from detailed interviews on a sample of almost 1000 successful ex-smokers. Very briefly, during **precontemplation** people do not feel impelled to do anything about their behaviour possibly due to ambivalence, denial, or selective exposure to information. As they become aware a problem exists they have entered the **contemplation** stage which is characterized by conflict and dissonance. The relatively brief **action** stage is when a commitment is made, while during **maintenance** new behaviour is strengthened. If **relapse** does not occur the individual eventually exits the change system to termination or in other words favourable long-term outcome. More recently, Di Clemente *et al.* (1991) have identified an additional stage called **preparation** between contemplation and action. Recent data (Prochaska *et al.* 1991) suggest that successful people do not necessarily progress in a linear fashion through the stages but they do nevertheless appear to pass through each stage at least once. Prochaska *et al.* (1992) would argue that these stages of change have been demonstrated across a variety of behaviours including alcohol and cocaine use, weight control, dieting and exercise.

The Prochaska and Di Clemente model is probably derivative and has been the subject of some criticism on both empirical and conceptual grounds (Davidson 1992). It has, on the other hand, been said to allow us to see things from a fresh perspective and casts the process of change in an entirely new mould (Orford 1992). Heather (1992) argues that the stages of change can now be reliably assessed and have considerable predictive validity. Evidence is also beginning to emerge (Prochaska *et al.* 1992) that various treatment interventions can be differentially effective at each stage.

CONCLUSIONS

This review has been selective and clearly there are other aspects of psychology which have a significant bearing on our understanding of personal change. The emphasis has been on the relationship between theory and practice and some of the work summarized has obvious application to our understanding of change in addictions. Perhaps the most immediately applicable is Brewin's (1988) attempt to provide an integrated framework for cognitive change processes based on experimental and social research.

Prior to his work, cognitive approaches to change variously emphasized attentional processes coping strategies, memory, and intentional appraisal. The only thing they appeared to have in common was a commitment to a cognitive mediational view of behaviour. Even Bandura's (1977) influential theory is not grounded on experimental research in cognitive processes and strategies. Brewin would acknowledge that his work does not formally take account of the social environment or a developmental perspective but rather concentrates on how people's knowledge of the world and themselves is stored, coded, accessed, and integrated with new experiences. His approach, however, could provide a theoretical rationale for the many cognitive change strategies currently employed by addiction workers and could help inform our sometimes arbitrary decisions on choice of intervention.

ACKNOWLEDGEMENTS

Special thanks to Rosemary Kent for her helpful comments on the first draft of this chapter.

REFERENCES

Abramson, L. Y., Seligman, M. E. P., and Teasdale, J. D. (1978). Learned helplessness in humans. Critique and reformulation. *Journal of Abnormal Psychology*, **87**, 49–74.

Annis, H. M. and Davis, C. S. (1989). Relapse prevention. In *Handbook of alcoholism treatment approaches: effective alternatives* (ed. R. K. Hester and W. R. Miller), pp. 170–82. Pergamon Press, New York.

Aranson, E. (1988). *The social animal*. Freeman, New York.

Asch, S. (1965). Effects of group pressure upon the modification and distortion of judgements. In *Basic studies in social psychology* (ed. H. Proshansky and B. Siedenberg), pp 230–52. Holt, Rinehart and Winston, New York.

Bandura, A. (1977). *Social learning theory*. Prentice-Hall, Englewood Cliffs, New Jersey.

Bandura, A. (1982). Self efficacy mechanism in human agency. *American Psychologist*, **37**, 122–47.

Beck, A. T. (1976). Cognitive therapy and the emotional disorders. International Universities Press, New York.

Becker, M. H. and Maiman, L. A. (1975). Sociobehavioural determinants of compliance with health and medical care recommendations. *Medical Care*, **13**, 10–24.

Bergin, A. E. (1980). Negative effects revised: a reply. *Professional Psychology*, **11**, 93–100.

Bibring, E. (1952). Psychoanalysis and the dynamic psychotherapies. *Journal American Psychoanalytic Association*, **2**, 745–70.

Block, J., Block, J. H., and Keyes, S. (1988). Longitudinally foretelling drug usage in adolescence: early childhood personality and environmental precursors. *Child Development*, **59**, 336–55.

Brewin, C. (1988). *Cognitive foundations of clinical psychology*. Erlbaum, Hillsdale.

Brewin, C. (1989). Cognitive change processes in psychotherapy. *Psychological Review*, **96**, 379–94.

Buller, P. F., Saxberg, B. O., and Smith, H. (1985). Institutionalisation of planned organisational change: a model and review of the literature. In *Developing human resources* (ed. L. Goodstein and J. W. Pfeiffer), pp. 189–99. University Associates, Oxford.

Cannon, D. S. and Baker, T. B. (1981). Emetic and electric shock alcohol aversion therapy: Assessment of conditioning. *Journal of Consulting Clinical Psychology*, **49**, 20–33.

Cannon, D. S., Baker, T. B., and Wehl, C. K. (1981). Emetic and electric shock alcohol aversion therapy: Six- and twelve-month follow-up. *Journal of Consulting Clinical Psychology*, **49**, 360–8.

Cheng, P. W. and Nowick, L. R. (1990). A probabilistic contrast model of causal induction. *Journal of Personality and Social Psychology*, **58**, 545–67.

Cialdine, R. (1988). *Influence: science and practice*. Harper Collins, New York.

Cross, W. E. (1971). The negro to black conversion experience: toward a psychology of black liberation. *Black World*, **20**, 13–27.

Davidson, R. (1991). Facilitating chance in problem drinkers. In *Counselling problem drinkers* (ed. R. Davidson, S. Rollnick, and I. MacEwan), pp. 3–20. Routledge, London.

Davidson, R. (1992). Prochaska and Di Clemente's model of change: a case study. *British Journal of Addiction*, **87**, 821–2.

Davies, J. B. (1992). *The myth of addiction*. Harwood Academic, Reading.

Diaz, R. M. and Fruhauf, A. G. (1991). The origins and development of self regulation. In *Self control and the addictive behaviours* (ed. N. Heather, W. Miller, and J. Greely). Maxwell Macmillan, New York.

Di Clemente, C. C., Prochaska, J. O., Fairhurst, S. K., Velicer, W. F., Velasquez, M. M., and Rossi, J. S. (1991). The processes of smoking cessation: an analysis of precontemplation, contemplation, and preparation stages of change. *Journal of Consulting and Clinical Psychology*, **59**, 295–304.

Dobson, K. S. (1988). *Handbook of cognitive-behavioral therapies*. Guilford Press, New York.

Dollard, J. and Miller, N. E. (1950). *Personality and psychotherapy*. McGraw-Hill, New York.

Donovan, D. and Chaney, E. (1985). Alcoholic relapse prevention and intervention. In *Relapse prevention: maintenance strategies in the treatment of addictive behaviours* (ed. G. Marlatt and J. Gordon), pp. 351–416.

Drummond, C., Cooper, T., and Glautier, S. (1990). Conditioned learning in alcohol dependence: implications for cue exposure treatment. *British Journal of Addiction*, **85**, 725–44.

D'Zurilla, T. and Goldfried, M. (1971). Problem solving and behaviour modification. *Journal of Abnormal Psychology*, **78**, 107–26.

Edwards, G. (1987). Book review of *Relapse prevention* (ed. C. A. Marlatt and J. R. Gordon). *British Journal of Addiction*, **82**, 319–23.

Edwards, G. (1994). Addiction, reductionism and Aaron's rod. *British Journal of Addiction*, **89**, 9–12.

Eiser, J. R. (1983). From attributions to behaviour. In *Attribution theory: social and functional extensions* (ed. M. Hewstone). Blackwell, Oxford.

Elkins, R. L. (1980). Covert sensitisation treatment of alcoholism: Contributions of successful conditioning to subsequent abstinence maintenance. *Addictive Behaviour*, **5**, 67–89.

Elkins, R. (1991). An appraisal of chemical aversion (emetic therapy) approaches to alcoholism treatment. *Behaviour Research and Therapy*, **29**, 387–413.

Ellis, A. (1962). *Reason and emotion in psychotherapy*. Lyle Stewart, New York.

English, H. and English, A. (1958). *Comprehensive dictionary of psychological and psychoanalytic terms*. McKay, New York.

Erikson, M. (1974). Forward to Watzlawick, P., Weakland, J. H., and Fisch, R. *Change principles of problem formation and problem resolution*. W. W. Norton & Co., New York.

Eysenck, H. J. (1987). Behaviour therapy and neurosis. In *Theoretical foundations of behaviour therapy* (ed. H. J. Eysenck and I. Martin), pp. 3–35. Plenum, New York.

Feather, N. T. (1982). *Expectations and actions: expectancy-value models in psychology*. N. J. Lawrence Erlbaum Associates Inc., Hillsdale.

Foa, E. B. and Kozak, M. J. (1986). Emotional processing of fear: Exposure to corrective information. *Psychological Bulletin*, **99**, 20–35.

Forsterling, F. (1985). Attributional retraining: a review. *Psychological Bulletin*, **98**, 495–512.

Garcia, J. (1989). Food for Tolman: Cognition and cathexis in concert. In *Aversion, Avoidance, and Anxiety: Perspectives on Aversively Motivated Behaviour* (ed. T. Acher and L. Nilsson), pp. 136–49. N. J. Erlbaum, Hillsdale.

Goldfried, M. R. (1980). Toward a delineation of therapeutic change principles. *American Psychologist*, **35**, 991–9.

Goldfried, M. R. and Robins, C. (1982). On the facilitation of self-efficacy. *Cognitive Therapy and Research*, **6**, 361–80.

Goldfried, M. and Safran, J. (1986). Future directions in psychotherapy integration. In *Handbook of Ecletic Psychotherapy* (ed. J. Norcross), pp.240–59. Brunner Mazel, New York.

Haney, C., Banks, C., and Zimbardo, P. (1973). Interpersonal dynamics in a simulated prison. *International Journal of Criminology and Penology*, **1**, 69–97.

Heather, N. (1992). Addictive disorders are essentially motivational problems. *British Journal of Addiction*, **87**, 828–30.

Heather, N. and Stallard, A. (1989). Does the Marlatt model underestimate the importance of conditioned craving in the relapse process? In *Relapse and addictive behaviour* (ed. M. Gossop). Routledge, Tavistock.

Heider, F. (1958). *The psychology of interpersonal relations*. Wiley, New York.

Hester, R. K. and Miller, W. R. (1989). *Handbook of Alcoholism treatment approaches: effective alternatives*. Pergamon Press, New York.

Hildebrand, P. (1983). The contemporary relevance of the psychodynamic tradition. In *Psychology and psychotherapy* (ed. D. Pilgrim), pp. 50–69. Routledge & Kegan Paul, London.

Janis, I. and Mann, L. (1977). *Decision-making: a psychological analysis of conflict, choice and commitment*. Free Press, New York.

Kanfer, F. H. (1986). Implications of a self-regulation model of therapy for treatment of addictive behaviours. In *Treating addictive behaviours: process of change* (ed. W. R. Miller and N. Heather), pp. 29–50. Plenum Press, New York.

Kanfer, F. H. and Grimm, G. L. (1980). Managing clinical change: a process model of therapy. *Behaviour Modification*, **4**, 419–44.

Keene, J. and Raynor, P. (1993). Addiction as a 'social weakness'. The influence of client and therapist beliefs. *Addiction Research*, **1**, 77–87.

Kelly, G. A. (1955). *The psychology of personal constructs*. Norton, New York.

Kelly, G. A. (1969). The psychotherapeutic relationship. In *Clinical psychology and personality: the selected papers of George Kelly* (ed. B. Maher). Wiley, New York.

Kelly, G. A. (1970). A brief introduction to personal construct theory. In *Perspectives in Personal Construct Theory*, (ed. D. Bannister). Academic Press, London.

Kirschenbaum, D. S. (1987). Self-regularity failure. A review with clinical implications. *Clinical Psychology Review*, **7**, 77–104.

Kohlberg, L. (1984). *The psychology of moral development: the nature and validity of moral stages*. Harper & Row, San Francisco.

Lafferty, P., Beutler, L. E., and Crago, M. (1989). Differences between more and less effective psychotherapists: a study of select therapist variables. *Journal of Consulting and Clinical Psychology*, **57**, 76–80.

Lambert, M. J., Dejulio, S. S., and Stein, D. M. (1978). Therapist interpersonal skills. Process, outcome, methodological considerations and recommendations for future research. *Psychological Bulletin*, **85**, 467–89.

Latimer, P. R. and Sweet, A. A. (1984). Cognitive vs. behavioural procedures in cognitive-behaviour therapy: a critical review of the evidence. *Journal of Behaviour Therapy and Experimental Psychiatry*, **15**, 9–22.

Lazarus, A. A. (1975). Multimodal behavioural therapy. In *Basic approaches to group psychotherapy and group counselling* (2nd edn) (ed. G. M. Gazda). Charles C. Thomas, Springfield, Illinois.

Levey, A. B. and Martin, I. (1987). Evaluative conditioning: a case for hedonic transfer. In *Theoretical foundations of behaviour therapy* (ed. H. J. Eysenck and I. Martin). Plenum Press, New York.

Lewin, K. (1947). Frontiers in group dynamics: concept, method and reality in social equilibrium and social change. *Human Relations*, **6**, 5–41.

Logue, A. W. (1985). Conditioned food aversion learning in humans. *Annals of the New York Academy of Sciences*, **443**, 316–29.

McCoy, M. M. (1981). Positive and negative emotion: a personal construct theory interpretation. In *Personal construct psychology: recent advances in theory and practice* (ed. H. Bonarius, R. Holland, and S. Rosenberg). Macmillan, London.

Mahoney, M. J. (1988). Constructive metatheory: I, basic features and historical foundations. *International Journal of Personal Construct Psychology*, **1**, 1–35.

Marks, I. M. (1987). *Fears, phobias and rituals: panic, anxiety and their disorders*. Oxford University Press, New York.

Markus, H. and Worf, E. (1987). The dynamic self-concept: a social psychological perspective. In *Annual review of psychology* (ed. M. R. Rosenzweig and L. W. Porter), pp. 73–81. CA Annual Reviews, Palo Alto.

Markus, H. R. and Kitayama, S. (1991). Culture and the self: implications for cognitive, emotion and motivation. *Psychological Review*, **98**, 224–53.

Marlatt, G. A. and Gordon, J. R. (1985). *Relapse prevention: maintenance strategies in the treatment of addictive behaviour*. Guilford Press, New York.

Marlatt, G. and Gordon, J. (1989). Relapse prevention: future directions. In *Relapse Prevention and Addictive Behaviour*, (ed. M. Gossop). Routledge, London.

Meichenbaum, D. (1977). *Cognitive behaviour modification*. Plenum, New York.

Meltzoff, J. and Kornreich, M. (1970). *Research on psychotherapy*. Atherton, New York.

Milgram, S. (1974). *Obedience to authority: an experimental view*. Harper and Row, New York.

Miller, W. R. and Baca, L. M. (1983). Two year follow-up of bibliotherapy and therapist-directed controlled drinking training for problem drinkers. *Behaviour Therapy*, **14**, 441–8.

Miller, W. and Rollnick, S. (1991). *Motivational Interviewing: Preparing people to change addictive behaviour*. Guilford, New York.

Nathan, P. E. (1985). Aversion therapy in the treatment of alcoholism: success and failure. *Annals of the New York Academy Sciences*, **443**, 357–64.

Orford, J. (1985). *Excessive appetites: a psychological view of addictions*. John Wiley, Chichester.

Orford, J. (1992). Davidson's dilemma. *British Journal of Addiction*, **27**, 832–3.

Papini, M. R. and Bitterman, M. E. (1990). The role of contingency in classical conditioning. *Psychological Review*, **97**, 396–403.

Parloff, M. B., London, P., and Wolfe, B. (1986). Individual psychotherapy and behaviour change. *Annual Review of Psychology*, **37**, 321–49.

Pentony, P. (1981). *Models of influence in psychotherapy*. Free Press, New York.

Phares, J. (1992). *Clinical psychology: concepts, methods and profession*. Brooks Cole, Pacific Grove.

Piorkowski, G. K. and Mann, E. T. (1975). Issues in treatment efficacy research with alcoholics. *Perceptual and Motor Skills*, **41**, 695–700.

Ponterotto, J. and Wise, S. (1987). Construct validity study of the Racial Identity Attitude Scale. *Journal of Counselling Psychology*, **14**, 218–23.

Powell, T., Bradley, B., and Gray, J. (1993). Subjective craving for opiates: evaluation of a cue exposure protocol for use with detoxified opiate addicts. *British Journal of Clinical Psychology*, **32**, 39–53.

Prochaska, J. O. (1979). *Systems of psychotherapy: a transtheoretical perspective*. Dorsey Press, Homewood, Ill.

Prochaska, J. O. and Di Clemente, C. C. (1983). Stages and processes of self-change of smoking: toward an integrated model of change. *Journal of Consulting Clinical Psychology*, **51**, 390–5.

Prochaska, J. O. and Di Clemente, C. C. (1984). *The transtheoretical approach: crossing traditional boundaries of therapy*. Dow-Jones Irwin, New York.

Prochaska, J. O., Velicer, W. F., Guadagnoli, E., Rossi, J. S., and Di Clemente, C. C. (1991). Patterns of change: dynamic typology applied to smoking cessation. *Multivariate Behavioural Research*, **26**, 83–107.

Prochaska, J., Di Clemente, C., Velicer, W., and Rossi, J. (1992). Criticisms and concerns of the transtheoretical model in light of recent research. *British Journal of Addiction*, **87**, 825–35.

Rachman, S. J. and Wilson, G. T. (1980). *The effects of psychological therapy* (2nd enlarged edn). Pergamon Press, New York.

Rescorla, R. (1988). Pavlovian conditioning: its not what you think. *American Psychologist*, **43**, 151–60.

Rogers, C. R. (1951). *Client-centred therapy*. Houghton Mifflin, Boston.

Rosenham, D. (1973). On being sane in insane places. *Science*, **179**, 250–8.

Rotter, J. B. (1975). Some problems and misconceptions related to the construct of internal versus external control of reinforcement. *Journal of Consulting and Clinical Psychology*, **43**, 56–67.

Rush, B. (1789). *Medical Inquiries and Observations*, Vol. 1. Griggs & Dickinsons, Philadelphia.

Ryle, A. (1984). How can we compare different psychotherapies? Why are they effective? *British Journal of Medical Psychology*, **57**, 261–4.

Saunders, B. and Allsop, S. (1991). Incentives and restraints: clinical research into problem drug use and self control. In *Self Control and the Addictive Behaviours* (ed. N. Heather, W. Miller, and J. Greely). Maxwell Macmillan, New York.

Saunders, W. M. and Kershaw, P. W. (1979). Spontaneous remission from alcoholism: a community study. *British Journal of Addiction*, **74**, 251–65.

Seligman, M. E. P. (1970). On the generality of the laws of learning. *Psychology Review*, **77**, 406–18.

Seligman, M. E. P. (1975). *Helplessness: on depression, development, and death*. Freeman, San Francisco.

Siegel, S. (1988). Drug anticipation and drug tolerance. In *Psychopharmacology of Addiction*, (ed. M. Lader). Oxford University Press, New York.

Smail, D. (1983). Psychotherapy and psychology. In *Psychology and psychotherapy*, (ed. D. Pilgrim), pp.7–20. Routledge & Kegan Paul, London.

Smith, D. (1982). Trends in counselling and psychotherapy. *American Psychologist*, **37**, 802–9.

Stewart, J. De Wit, H. and Eikelboom, R. (1984). Role of unconditioned and conditioned drug effects in the self administration of opiates and stimulants. *Psychological Review*, **91**, 251–68.

Stockwell, T. (1992). Models of change, heavenly bodies and weltanschauugs. *British Journal of Addiction*, **87**, 830–1.

Takens, R. J. (1987). Personal construct theory and client-centred therapy: two sides of a coin. Paper presented at 7th International Congress on Personal Construct Psychology, Memphis.

Tolman, E. C. (1948). Cognitive maps in rats and men. *Psychological Review*, **55**, 189–208.

Truax, C. B. and Mitchell, K. M. (1971). Research on certain therapist interpersonal skills in relation to process and outcome. In *Handbook of psychotherapy and behaviour change: an empirical analysis* (ed. A. E. Bergin, S. L. Garfield). Wiley, New York.

Tuchfeld, B. (1976). Changes in the patterns of alcohol use without the aid of formal treatment. *Research Triangle Institute*, North Carolina.

Wachtel, P. L. (1977). *Psychoanalysis and behaviour therapy. Toward an integration*. Basic Books, New York.

Wade, C. and Tavris, C. (1993). *Psychology*. Harper Collins, New York.

Watzlawick, P., Weakland, J. H., and Fisch, R. (1974). *Change principles of problem formation and problem resolution*. W. W. Norton & Co., New York.

Weiner, B. (1985). An attributional theory of achievement motivation and emotion. *Psychological Review*, **92**, 548–73.

Weiner, B. (1986). *An attributional theory of motivation and emotion*. Springer-Verlag, New York.

Wertsch, J. V. (1984). The zone of proximal development: some conceptual issues. In *Children's learning in the zone of proximal development* (ed. B. Rocoff and J. V. Wertsch). C. A. Jossey-Bass.

Wessells, M. G. (1982). *Cognitive psychology*. Harper & Row, New York.

Wikler, A. (1965). Conditioning factors in opiate addiction and relapse. In *Narcotics* (ed. D. Wiher and G. Kissebaum). McGraw-Hill, New York.

Wilson, T. (1991). Chemical aversion conditioning in the treatment of alcoholism: further comments. *Behaviour Research and Therapy*, **29**, 415–19.

Winter, D. (1992). *Personal Construct Psychology in Clinical Practice*. Routledge, London.

5

Dependence and the correlates of change: a review of the literature

REGINALD G. SMART

Most of us would agree with Babor (1990) that there has never been a 'clear cut, universally accepted definition of dependence'. Rather there has been a proliferation of definitions suggested by individuals, committees, learned societies, and international organizations. Of course, this makes any effort to look at the correlates of change in dependency more difficult. Most investigators seem to hold a definition which combines both psychological and physical attributes, perhaps similar to the WHO (1978) definition:

A state, psychic and usually also physical, resulting from taking alcohol, characterized by behavioural and other responses that always include a compulsion to take alcohol on a continuous or periodic basis in order to experience its psychic effects, and sometimes to avoid the discomfort of its absence; tolerance may or may not be present (WHO 1978).

Several additional problems arise when we try to look at the correlates of change in dependence. One problem is that there is no clearly defined set of researchers having that as their main activity, and no single journal focus for the research. There are many studies with various other agendas that focus some attention on the correlates of change in dependence. These include studies of the natural history of addiction, longitudinal studies, efforts to look at treatment and spontaneous recovery, and studies of addict characteristics. Altogether, the material presents a mixed and somewhat incomplete picture. Probably our picture of the correlates of decreased dependence is better than our picture of why people increase their dependence on drugs. Four major questions we can ask are:

1. Is there a natural progression for dependence?

2. What are the correlates of increased dependence or its initiation?

3. What are the correlates of relapses to dependence from abstinence?

4. What are the correlates of decreased dependence or a total return to normal?

In this review treatment outcome studies have largely been excluded and the focus is instead on the other correlates of change in dependence. Treatment outcome studies have often been reviewed before (Miller and Hester 1986; Ogborne 1978).

IS THERE A NATURAL PROGRESSION IN DEPENDENCE?

The idea that there is a natural progression over time for the symptoms underlying alcohol and drug dependence is an old one. Jellinek's phases of addiction study in 1946 (Jellinek 1952) first set out the idea that alcoholism was a progressive disease and that there was an inexorable progression towards abstinence or death. His original research on the order in which symptoms arose in alcoholics was based on a study of Alcoholics Anonymous members. It became part of the early mythology of alcoholism and was greatly admired by Alcoholics Anonymous and many of those who first worked in alcoholism treatment centres.

Despite the simplicity and attractiveness of the 'phases' approach no one has been able to duplicate Jellinek's results in the detail he presented. Park and Whitehead (1973), for example, studied the symptoms progression for 806 alcoholics. They found that for 28 of 43 Jellinek items there was a determinable order but that order was different to that found by Jellinek. Since that study many researchers have failed to find the expected progression. Clark and Cahalan (1976) studied 52 problem drinking men at two intervals four years apart. Loss of control at time one correlated only 0.13 with loss of control at time two, although some alcoholics with severe problems had died. Also, 18 of 29 binge drinkers reported no loss of control. Ojesjo (1981) studied 96 alcoholics twice at 15-year intervals and found considerable shifting amongst major drinking categories. For example, of 29 classed as alcohol dependent in 1957 only eight were still in that category 15 years later. Of the 49 alcohol abusers in 1957, 17 became chronic alcoholics or died.

Vaillant (1983) claimed that progression is not found in some studies of alcohol abusers because:

1. Many chronic alcoholics die and are left out of the later phases of longitudinal studies.

2. Some studies used problem drinkers rather than later or end-stage alcoholics.

Several people (Trice and Wahl 1958; Horn and Wanberg 1969; Vaillant 1983) have found some general support for the phases proposed by Jellinek, while not agreeing on every symptom or its developmental placement. In general, blackouts and frequent intoxication come first, then complaints by significant others, then loss of control and attempts to stop drinking, followed by benders, alcoholic hallucinosis, and delirium tremens. There are, however, many atypical alcoholics and considerable shifting back and forth between abstinence and serious symptoms of alcoholism.

Fillmore's (1987) longitudinal studies have shown that problem drinking and social complications are more common among the youth, and that they decrease and stabilize in middle age before dropping in the sixties. Fillmore acknowledges that sample attrition and mortality account for some of the results but claims that their effects are minimal. Her latest analysis of 27 longitudinal data sets from many countries showed that declines in consumption with age were common, however, individual level findings were less homogeneous (Fillmore *et al.* 1991).

The idea of a natural progression over time has also been prevalent as an explanation of drug abuse. Winick (1962) was one of the first to suggest that drug addicts (chiefly heroin addicts) would 'mature out' of their addiction at around age 40. This was seen as a natural part of the passage of time and some other vague factors. No specific ordering of factors was given, but Winick's theory made reference to better psychological insight and increased pressure from law enforcement as important influences on addicts. Winick based his research on arrest files which showed that heroin addicts were less frequently arrested after the age of 40.

Little research has been focused directly on the maturing out theory. Ball and Snarr (1969) found that criminality increased among addicted males in Puerto Rico but decreased among those who become abstinent. About 20–40 per cent of opiate addicts treated at Lexington became abstinent by age 40. Snow (1973) also found that 23 per cent of addicts on a New York City register became abstinent by age 40. Limited support is available for the maturing out theory.

Research on the natural progression of dependence involving 'phases' or 'maturing out' seems to have largely disappeared and the concepts are no longer fashionable. However, neither concept has been sufficiently explored. Research interests have recently turned toward factors or correlates of change in alcohol and drug dependence and problems.

WHAT ARE THE CORRELATES OF ESCALATION TO DEPENDENCE?

Surprisingly few research projects have focused on how dependence increases and far more has been done on how dependence ends. Most of what is known about how dependence increases comes from retrospective studies of addicts recounting memories of how they started to be dependent. Some information is available about how increased drug use and availability, psychological problems and changes in social stability relate to increased dependence.

The natural history of drug addiction can be organized into various phases as few people become dependent with their first drink or drug use. Waldorf (1983) has suggested six phases including:

1. Experimentation or initiation; most users stop at this stage.

2. Escalation: an increase in use up to daily use; later stages include withdrawal symptoms, tolerance, and other symptoms of dependency.

3. Maintaining or 'taking care of business'; a period of stable drug use, maintaining supplies and the habit.

4. Dysfunction or 'going through changes'; characterized by attempts to stop drug use, obtain treatment, and experiences of jail.

5. Recovery or 'getting out of the life': the drug user makes an effort to stop using drugs, gives up drug-using friends and may move away,

6. Ex-addict: a phase in which ex-addicts develop a social identity around their former habit. They may go to work in treatment programs.

Despite the general acceptance of a natural history of dependence, research on the correlates of movement from experimentation to escalation and dependency is often fragmentary and contradictory. Some information does exist on the role of increased drug use, availability, psychological problems, and social stability.

Increases in drug use

We would expect that movement from experimentation or social drinking into dependence would be accompanied by changes in the amount or pattern of use. Only a few studies have been made on the topic. Sanchez-Craig and Israel (1985) studied 70 problem drinkers who were relatively young (around age 35) and not yet at the 'alcoholic' stage. They found that when alcohol consumption exceeded four drinks on three days per week problems developed, but below that level there were few problems. This study suggests a limit for movement from experimentation to escalation, but it does not establish a limit for moving into dependency. Horn and Wanberg (1968) in their study of hospitalized alcoholics found evidence that beer drinking was associated with an early, relatively problem-free stage and that spirits drinking was associated with a transition into dependency.

Unfortunately, we have little empirical work on how an increased use of drugs such as opiates, barbiturates, or cocaine relates to the movement into dependence. Much clinical experience and some natural history studies (Waldorf and Biernacki 1979; Robins and Murphy 1973) suggest that daily use of such drugs leads to dependency, but some drug users seem able to use daily for short periods with no dependency (Zinberg 1979).

Availability

The single distribution theory developed by Popham *et al.* (1976) of alcohol consumption, argued that overall per capita alcohol consumption and heavy consumption and cirrhosis were related. This theory also contained the notion that the best way for governments to control heavy consumption was to reduce alcohol availability and hold overall consumption down. The theory was not meant to predict changes at the level of individual drinkers but it could have been used in that way.

Availability as a factor in consumption has been more important in research on illicit drugs. Many studies have shown that the movement of users into heavy drug use and perhaps dependency is associated with increased availability of drugs. For example, Simpson *et al.* (1986), in their 12-year follow-up study of opiate addicts, found that the availability of opiates was very or somewhat important for 73 per cent of addicts in starting daily opiate use. However, it was less important than psychological factors such as anxiety reduction, sensation seeking, and the desire to have 'the rush'. Barrett *et al.* (1990) using the same sample as Simpson found that drug availability was perceived as important at several transition stages—starting and stopping daily opiate use. However, it was perceived by addicts as more important when beginning addiction. Kandel (1984) also reported that adult frequent marihuana users more often found it easy or very easy to get than did less frequent users.

Some informal evidence that increased availability leads to cocaine dependence is found in the 11-year follow-up of cocaine users reported by Murphy *et al*. (1989). Several of the users did develop problems and dependency. In all cases there was increased access to cocaine because relatives began dealing it or because a large inheritance made more money available.

The most striking instance of increased drug availability leading to dependency probably occurred during the Vietnam War. Large numbers of young soldiers were suddenly exposed to cheap, high-quality opiates and other drugs at a time when many were prone to drug use and felt they needed it for psychological reasons. Robins' (1973) study of the Vietnam Veteran has been a classic in the literature, showing how important increased availability can be. Robins (1973) found that about 9.5 per cent of all enlisted men were dependent on drugs on leaving Vietnam. However, very few of those who became dependent had ever tried heroin before going to Vietnam. The best predictors of narcotic use in Vietnam were pre-service drug use, multiple drug use, heavy drinking, delinquency, being under age 20, and being an enlistee rather than a draftee. Probably the increased drug use was related to increased availability but also to the need to deal with the boredom and the anxiety associated with wartime service.

Increased psychological problems

Many investigators have found that alcoholics and drug addicts have some psychological problems before their dependency (Robins and Murphy 1973; Vaillant 1983; Shedler and Block 1990) usually sociopathic personality or depression. The difference between essential and reactive alcoholism, especially among women has been long been recognized. It is plausible that increases in anxiety, depression, or other psychological problems could lead to increased drug use and a movement into dependency. However, I have been able to find very little empirical research confirming that progression. Simpson *et al*. (1986) found that addicts most often gave sensation seeking and anxiety reduction as the reasons why they started daily opiate use. Vaillant (1983) has reviewed the evidence that depression and alcoholism are related and from this review and his own work has concluded that depression follows alcoholism not vice versa. Many studies have shown that drug addicts are depressed (Woody and Blaine 1979). However, we have no direct evidence that increases in depression lead to a movement into dependency on any drug, although the proposition does seem plausible.

On a more general societal level there is limited evidence that drinking and depression are related. Hartka *et al.'s* (1991) meta-analysis of eight longitudinal studies in four countries showed that early depression predicted later consumption among females but not males.

Changes in social stability

Numerous studies (Robins 1973; Dupont *et al.* 1979; Vaillant 1983) show that American drug abusers, especially opiate addicts are more likely to come from lower class, ghetto backgrounds with unstable family histories. This literature is too large to review here. Little direct evidence can be found that decreases in social stability such as unemployment, loss of spouse or other family members leads from escalation to dependence. Yamaguchi and Kandel (1985) have found that marihuana use, especially heavy use, leads to the postponement of marriage. Marriage leads to stopping marihuana use for women (but not men).

WHAT ARE THE CORRELATES OF RELAPSES TO DEPENDENCY FROM ABSTINENCE?

It is well known that both alcoholics and drug abusers have a high rate of relapse from successful treatment. Relapse rates vary greatly, but can be as high as 90 per cent (Ogborne 1978; Miller and Hester 1986). Considerable research has been done on the reasons for relapses for alcohol and opiate dependency by Marlatt and his colleagues. For example, Cummings *et al.* (1980) found that 71 per cent of alcoholic relapses were related to three high-risk situations,

1. negative emotional states such as anger or depression;

2. conflict, argument, or unpleasant exchanges with others;

3. pressures from other people, whether direct or not, to drink alcohol.

This research showed that physiological reasons were not the primary reasons for relapse and has led to considerable research on relapse prevention methods (Marlatt and Gordon 1985; George 1989; Annis 1990).

Annis (1990) has developed a model of relapse prevention and has found that different clients have different relapse patterns. She developed an Inventory of Drinking Situations (IDS) which gives drinking risk scores in terms of unpleasant emotions, physical discomfort, pleasant emotions, testing personal control, urges and temptations, conflict with others, social pressures to drink, and good times with others. About 88 per cent of alcoholics seeking treatment at the Addiction Research Foundation in Toronto had one of four profiles:

1. high negative (24 per cent), more drinking after unpleasant emotions and conflict with others;

2. high positive (8 per cent), more drinking in response to pleasant emotions and pressures to drink;

3. low physical discomfort (30 per cent), less drinking in response to physical discomfort than other groups;

4. low testing personal controls (26 per cent) less drinking in response to testing controls.

Alcoholics with a high negative profile were more likely to drink alone, have a higher level of alcohol dependence, and to be female. Those with a high positive profile were more likely to drink with others, have lower alcohol dependence scores, and to be male. Other differentiations were less reliable.

The Marlatt and Annis approaches to relapse prevention have also been used in research on opiate and cocaine dependency. For example, Bradley *et al.* (1989) used the Cummings and Marlatt approach in a study of relapse to opiate use following detoxification. About two-thirds of those who relapsed did so after making an explicit plan to try opiates again in a controlled way. About half said that negative mood states such as sadness, loneliness, boredom, tension and anxiety led to the relapse. Unlike Marlatt, Bradley *et al.* did not find that social pressures to use drugs were important. This may be due in part to how they asked questions of addicts and their emphasis on cognitive factors, an area not much investigated by Marlatt.

The role of substance abuse or use cues in triggering relapse remains controversial. This involves cues such as seeing the drugs or paraphernalia or being in drug coping areas. However, Bradley *et al.* (1989) found that craving and drug-related cues were relatively unimportant in relapses.

A study by Heather *et al.* (1991) showed that temptations or urges in the presence of substance cues were not important in relapse when ratings were made of open-ended addict responses by judges. However, they were the most important reason given by heroin addicts. What explanation could be given for these conflicting results is unclear. Bradley *et al.* (1986) used opiate addicts from London, and Heather *et al.* used heroin addicts from London, Dundee, and Sydney. Probably, much of the problem could be explained by the different lists of relapse possibilities presented to addicts.

Much relapse research has been done on Marlatt's category of negative emotional states. For example, Rhoads (1983) and Judson and Goldstein (1983) found that heroin addicts relapsed mainly because of negative emotional states and lack of social supports. Kosten *et al.* (1986) also found that relapsed heroin addicts had more negative life experiences post-treatment and more depression at intake. However, a recent study by Hall *et al.* (1991) of relapse for cocaine addicts found rather different results. Cocaine addicts who endorsed a total abstinence goal were very unlikely to relapse. Mood scores were obtained for the weeks prior to relapse. Positive moods predicted a lower risk of relapse but negative moods, hassles, and life events were not associated with relapses. Clearly much work remains to be done on predictors of relapse, especially combining pretreatment variables, treatment process variables/and post-treatment factors.

WHAT ARE THE CORRELATES OF DECREASED DEPENDENCE?

Much interest has been taken in the correlates of decreased dependence. There are studies of recovery without treatment for both alcoholics and addicts as well as a variety of longitudinal studies examining why drug-dependent persons have improved. The main factors seem to be burn-out or addict fatigue, better personal willpower and motivation, changes in the environment, physical or psychological problems, religious conversion, and changes in social stability. Many addicts and alcoholics, of course, report several reasons.

Burn-out and addict fatigue

Street level addicts to drugs such as opiates and cocaine live difficult, exhausting, and punishing lives. Eventually most seem to get into trouble with the law or their families and many develop physical problems. Waldorf (1983) has summarized many studies on the socio-psychological aspects of recovery for addicts, and burn-out is a common feature. In many cases addicts seem to burn-out due to the combined difficulties of the addict lifestyle and pressures from the judicial system. Vaillant (1973) showed that addicts who were given parole and mandatory supervision were more likely to become abstinent than those who did not. In the study by Simpson *et al.* (1986) the most important reasons for addicts quitting daily opioid use were that they were tired of 'the hustle' and 'needed a change' (hit bottom).

Klingemann's study (1990) of 'remitters' from heroin and alcohol addiction also showed the importance of negative events and hitting bottom. A majority mentioned negative events such as health, jobs, and financial problems, as well as feelings of helplessness and insecurity, family tensions, and trouble with the police in the year prior to 're-mitting'. Smaller numbers mentioned positive events such as moving, starting school, and job improvements. He has shown that there are many who are motivated by hitting bottom and a smaller number of self-changers and people who respond to positive changes. One almost unique feature of the Klingemann study is that it obtained information from collaterals.

One aspect of 'burn-out' seems to be an increase in 'humiliating experiences' such as an experience in jail, ridicule or rejection by a friend, or embarrassment in front of children or other relatives. Waldorf (1983) found this to be the most often reported motivation for addicts to stop using opiates; 44 per cent reported it. Tuchfeld (1981), in his study of spontaneous recovery in alcoholics, also found that humiliating experiences were the most important factor.

Reported personal motivation

Much has been written about 'spontaneous recovery' or recovery without treatment (Smart 1975; Tuchfeld *et al.* 1976; Vaillant 1983), yearly rates varying from 1 to 33 per cent depending on the study. On close examination many social and personal factors are involved in 'spontaneous' recovery. Several studies have indicated that drug dependents sometimes make the simple decision to stop using, with few outside influences. For example, Waldorf (1983) found that the most important reason given by addicts was 'it was time to do other things' (29 per cent) or I had 'no alternative but to quit'. In Vaillant's study about half of the abstinent men attributed their abstinence to 'willpower'. Tuchfeld (1981) found that alcoholics in his study were proud of their ability to resolve their alcohol problems on their own. Many had quit smoking previously and saw themselves as strong-willed, determined people.

Negative life events seemed to be the most common experiences enabling alcoholics to abstain in the study by Edwards *et al.* (1992) although 'Damascus' or sudden insight experiences seemingly unmoti-vated were also common. Sometimes alcoholics and drug abusers just seem to decide to stop. Jorquez (1983) also found that heroin addicts who stopped often had profound cognitive and emotional experiences during crisis episodes. They had longer struggles to extricate themselves from addict lifestyles and accommodate themselves to a 'square' existence. Of course most studies of personal motivation take at face value what the former alcoholic or drug user says about it. If we had more collateral reports from spouses, employers or friends, our picture would be more complete.

Environmental changes

Many believe that addicts and alcoholics cannot solve their problems without a change in their environment which in turn promotes a drug-free lifestyle. Maddux and Desmond (1980) and Schasre (1966) reported that addicts who did well after treatment cited relocation from their usual drug sources and decreased drug supplies as the major factor in recovery. Waldorf (1983) also found that once addicts decide to quit they have to give up old friends, avoid drug using situations, and develop leisure or recreational interests to be successful.

As mentioned earlier Robins' study (1973) of Vietnam Veterans clearly showed the effect of environment on dependency. Of the veterans who tested positive for narcotics when they left Vietnam only 8 per cent were using narcotics at the time of the follow-up interview and only 5 per cent had been treated for a drug problem. Those who continued using after returning had more often used before Vietnam and used heavily when there. This study gives evidence of a startling remission rate when drug availability and the need to use drugs are reduced.

Physical or psychological problems

Several studies have reported that physical or psychological problems were important in recovery. Maddux and Desmond (1980) found that many abstinent addicts had 'rock bottom' experiences after repeated illnesses or imprisonment. In Waldorf's (1983) study only 23.9 per cent of addicts reported that personal health problems were important in helping them stop opiate use. Also, in Frykholm's study (1985) only a quarter of addicts gave adverse drug effects or complications as the main reason for giving up drugs. Some others gave adverse effects as a contributing factor but 'burn-out' was the main one cited. Some spontaneous recovery studies among alcoholics have also mentioned health concerns (Saunders and Kershaw 1979; Tuchfield 1981) but they do not seem to be the most important factors.

Vaillant's long-term study of alcoholics (1983) provides the greatest support for health factors. About half of Vaillant's alcoholics who were 'securely abstinent' mentioned medical consequences as an important factor in securing it. In all of these studies, however, multiple reasons were given and the possible reasons vary considerably from one study to another. No two studies have exactly the same answer categories so detailed comparisons cannot be made. Not much research is available on how decreased psychological problems such as depression or anxiety relate to decreased dependency, except for Vaillant's study which shows that depression does not lead to alcoholism.

Religious Experiences

Religious experiences often precede or coincide with the decision to decrease alcohol or drug use. Alcoholics Anonymous can be seen as a religious-based self-help group as the alcoholic agrees to recognize some higher power. Of course many people recover through AA, but it is not clear how important the religious aspect is in recovery. Religious experiences are mentioned as a factor in the Tuchfield (1981) study, but they are given little prominence. Also, only two of 58 addicts in Frykholm's (1985) study mentioned such experiences as a main or contributory factor. Vaillant found that only 12 per cent of alcoholics named religion as a factor in abstinence. However, Waldorf (1983) asked about religious experience and spiritual experience separately as factors in recovery. More addicts mentioned 'spiritual' experiences (21.1 per cent) than 'religious' experiences (15.5 per cent), but together these categories include nearly half of the opiate addicts.

Social stability

It should be expected that a sudden or gradual increase in social stability could lead to decreased drug dependence. This might include marriage or a new relationship, getting a job or completing schooling. Several studies have shown that both alcoholics (Edwards *et al.* 1992) and drug addicts (Waldorf 1983; Frykholm 1985; Simpson *et al.* 1986) may respond to increased pressure from spouses or children. In the Simpson *et al.* study, 54 per cent stated family responsibility and 17 per cent divorce or separation as being very important or somewhat important in helping them quit opiate use. About 25 per cent thought obtaining a new or better job was most important and 21 per cent mentioned fear of losing a job. Also, 55 per cent of those who recovered without treatment reported having a new spouse or new relationship during recovery.

Some complex relationships between social stability and quitting marihuana use have been found by Yamaguchi and Kandel (1985) in their study of adults. Marriage led to stopping marihuana use for women, while parenthood, but not marriage alone, led to stopping marihuana use for men. They also found a close correlation between the use of illicit drugs and premarital cohabitation.

Of course, marriage, especially to a heavy drug user, may promote drug use. Several abusers have noted (for example Brill 1972; Waldorf 1983) that there is situational addiction by spouses, especially women living with drug addicts. Their drug use often ends when the relationship ends.

THE RESEARCH FUTURE

In summary, research on the correlates of change in dependence is diffuse and rather incomplete. We have less information on escalation to dependence than we have for decreased dependence or relapses from abstinence. In all types of change, availability and personal motivation seem to be important. Factors such as psychological problems, social stability, and religious experiences are not clearly established as important factors for most dependent persons. However, in some instances they seem to be crucially important.

The research literature still has a number of problems. Nearly all the research depends upon retrospective accounts by drug or alcohol users on the reasons why their dependency level changed. There apparently are no direct observational studies and few studies use information from collaterals. We are left, then, with some questions about how these accounts are affected by memory loss, social desirability, and other factors. An additional problem has been that no two investigators examine the same reasons for change or even ask the questions in a similar way. The closest correspondence seems to be for researchers using Marlatt's theories of relapse. In general, the field could do with more standardization of measurement and less exclusive use of retrospective accounts.

REFERENCES

Annis, J. M. (1990). Relapse to substance abuse: empirical findings within a cognitive-social learning approach. *Journal of Psychoactive Drugs*, **22**, 117–24.

Babor, T. (1990). Social, scientific and medical issues in the definition of alcohol and drug dependence. In *The nature of drug dependence* (ed. G. Edwards and M. Lader), pp. 19–35. Oxford University Press.

Ball, J. C. and Snarr, R. W. (1969). A test of the maturation hypothesis with respect to opiate addiction. *Bulletin of Narcotics*, **21**, 9–13.

Barrett, M. E., Joe, G. W., and Simpson, D. D. (1990). Availability of drugs and psychological proneness in opioid addiction. *International Journal of Addictions*, **25**, 1211–26.

Bradley, G. P., Phillips, G., Green, L., and Gossop, M. (1989). Circumstances surrounding initial relapse to opiate use following detoxification. *British Journal of Psychiatry*, **154**, 354–9.

Brill, L. (1972). *The re-addiction process*. Charles C. Thomas, Springfield.

Clark, W. B. and Cahalan, D. (1976). Changes in problem drinking over a four-year span. *Addictive Behaviors*, **1**, 251–9.

Cummings, C., Gordon, J. R., and Marlatt, G. A. (1980). Relapse: Prevention and prediction. In *The addictive behaviors: treatment of alcoholism, drug abuse, smoking and obesity* (ed. W. R. Miller), pp. 291–381. Pergamon, New York.

Dupont, R. L., Goldstein, A., and O'Donnell, J. (1979). *Handbook on drug abuse*. National Institute on Drug Abuse, Washington.

Edwards, G., Oppenheimer, E., and Taylor, C. (1992). Hearing the noise in the system: exploration of textual analysis as a method for studying change in drinking behaviour. *British Journal of Addiction*, **87**, 73–81.

Fillmore, K. M. (1987). Prevalence, incidence and chronicity of drinking patterns and problems among men as a function of age: a longitudinal and cohort analysis. *British Journal of Addiction*, **82**, 77–83.

Fillmore, K. M., Hartka, E., Johnstone, B. M., Leino, V., Motoyoski, M., and Temple, M. T. (1991). A meta-analysis of life course variation in drinking. *British Journal of Addiction*, **86**, 1221–68.

Frykholm, B. (1985). The drug career. *Journal of Drug Issues*, **15**, 333–46.

George, W. H. (1989). Marlatt and Gordon's relapse prevention model: a cognitive—behavioral approach to understanding and preventing relapse. *Journal of Chemical Dependency Treatment*, **2**, 125–52.

Hall, S. M., Harassy, B. E., and Wauseman, D. A. (1991). Effects of commitment to abstinence, positive moods, stress and coping on relapse to cocaine use. *Journal of Consulting and Clinical Psychology*, **59**, 526–32.

Hartka, E., Johnston, B., Leino, E. V., Motoyoski, M., Temple, M. T., and Fillmore, K. M. (1991). A meta-analysis of depressive symptomatology and alcohol consumption over time. *British Journal of Addiction*, **86**, 1283–98.

Heather, N., Stallard, A., and Tebutt, J. (1991). Importance of substance abuse cues in relapse among heroin users: comparison of two methods of investigation. *Addictive Behaviours*, **16**, 41–9.

Horn, J. L. and Wanberg, K. W. (1969). Symptom patterns related to excessive use of alcohol. *Journal of Studies on Alcohol*, **30**, 35–58.

Jellinek, E. M. (1952). Phases of Alcohol Addiction. *Quarterly Journal of Studies on Alcohol*, **13**, 673–84.

Jorquez, J. S. (1983). The retirement phase of heroin using careers. *Journal of Drug Issues*, **13**, 343–65.

Judson, B. A. and Goldstein, A. (1983). Episodes of heroin use during maintenance treatment with a stable dosage of α—acetyl—methadol. *Drug and Alcohol Dependence*, **11**, 271–8.

Kandel, D. B. (1984). Marihuana uses in young adulthood. *Archives of General Psychiatry*, **41**, 200–9.

Klingemann, H. H. (1990). 'Hitting rock bottom' or 'the power of the positive' —motivational forces towards the recovery from problematic alcohol and heroin use. Paper presented at Kettil Bruun Society Meeting, Budapest, 1990.

Kosten, T. R., Rounsville, B. J., and Kleber, H. D. (1986). A 2.5 year follow up of depression, life crises and treatment effects on abstinence among opioid addicts. *Archives of General Psychiatry*, **43**, 733–8.

Maddux, J. F. and Desmond, D. P. (1980). New light on the maturing out hypothesis in opioid dependence. *Bulletin on Narcotics*, **32**, 15–25.

Marlatt, G. A. and Gordon, J. R. (1985). *Relapse prevention: maintenance strategies in the treatment of addictive behaviours*. Guilford Press, Guilford.

Miller, W. R. and Hester, R. R. (1986). The effectiveness of alcoholism treatment: what research reveals. In *The addictive behaviors: treatment of alcoholism, drug abuse, smoking and obesity* (ed. W. R. Miller and N. Heather), pp. 121–74. Pergamon, New York.

Murphy, S., Reinarman, C., and Waldorf, D. (1989). An 11 year follow-up of a network of cocaine users. *British Journal of Addiction*, **84**, 427–36.

Ogborne, A. (1978). Patient characteristics as predictors of treatment outcomes for alcohol and drug abusers. In *Research advances in alcohol and drug problems* (ed. Y. Israel, F. Glaser, H. Kalant, R. E. Popham, W. Schmidt, and R. Smart), pp. 177–224. Plenum, Toronto.

Ojesjo, L. (1981). Long-term outcome in alcohol abuse and alcoholism among males in the Lundby general population, Sweden. *British Journal of Addiction*, **76**, 391–400.

Park, P. and Whitehead, P. C. (1973). Developmental sequence and dimensions of alcoholism. *Quarterly Journal on Studies on Alcohol*, **34**, 887–904.

Popham, R. E., Schmidt, W., and de Lint, J. (1976). The effects of legal restraint on drinking. In *The biology of alcoholism*, Vol. 4 (ed. B. Kissin and H. Begleiter), pp. 579–625. Plenum, New York.

Rhoads, D. (1983). A longitudinal study of life stress and social support among drug abusers. *International Journal of Addictions*, **18**, 195–222.

Robins, L. N. (1973). *The Vietnam Drug User Returns*, US Government Printing Office, Washington, DC.

Robins, L. N. and Murphy, G. T. (1973). Drug use in a normal population of young negro men. *American Journal of Public Health*, **67**, 57(9).

Sanchez-Craig, M. and Israel, Y. (1985). Pattern of alcohol use associated with self-identified problem drinking. *American Journal of Public Health*, **75**, 178–80.

Saunders, W. M. and Kershaw, P. W. (1979). Spontaneous remission from alcoholism—a community study. *British Journal of Addiction*, **74**, 251–66.

Schasre, R. (1966). Cessation patterns among neophyte heroin users. *International Journal of Addictions*, **1**, 23–32.

Shedler, J. and Block, J. (1990). Adolescent drug use and psychological health: a longitudinal inquiry. *American Psychologist*, **45**, 612–30.

Simpson, D. D., Joe, G. W., Lehman, W. E., and Sells, S. B. (1986). Addiction careers: etiology, treatment and 12 year follow-up outcomes. *Journal of Drug Issues*, **16**, 107–21.

Smart, R. G. (1975). Spontaneous recovery in alcoholics: a review and analysis of the available research (1975). *Drug and Alcohol Dependence*, **1**, 277–85.

Snow, M. (1973). Maturing out of narcotic addiction in New York City. *International Journal of Addictions*, **8**, 921–38.

Trice, H. M. and Wahl, J. R. (1958). A rank order analysis of the symptoms of alcoholism. *Quarterly Journal on Studies on Alcohol*, **19**, 636–48.

Tuchfeld, B. S., Simuel, J. B., Schmitt, Ries, J. L., Ray, D., and Waterhouse, G. J. (1976). Changes in patterns of alcohol use without the aid of formal treatment: an exploratory study of former drinkers. Contract ADM 281–750–0023, Research Triangle Institute, Research Triangle Park, North Carolina.

Vaillant G. E. (1973). A 20 year follow-up of New York narcotic adults. *Archives of General Psychiatry*, **29**, 237–41.

Vaillant G. E. (1983). *The natural history of alcoholism*. Harvard University Press, Cambridge.

Waldorf, D. and Biernacki, P. (1979). Natural recovery from heroin addiction: a review of the incidence literature. *Journal of Drug Issues*, **9**, 281–9.

Waldorf, D. (1983). Natural recovery from opiate addiction: Some social-psychological processes of untreated recovery. *Journal of Drug Issues*, **13**, 237–80.

Winick, C. (1962). Maturing out of narcotic addiction. *Bulletin on Narcotics*, **13**, 1–8.

Woody, G. E. and Blaine, J. (1979). Depression in narcotic addicts: quite possibly more than a chance association. In *Handbook on drug abuse* (ed. R. L. Dupont, A. Goldstein, and J. O'Donnell), pp. 277–85. National Institute on Drug Abuse, Washington.

World Health Organization (1978). *Mental disorders: glossary and guide to their classification in accordance with the ninth revision of the international classification of diseases*. World Health Organization, Geneva.

Yamaguchi, K. and Kandel, D. B. (1985). Dynamic relationships between pre-marital cohabitation and illicit drug use: an event-history analysis of role selection and role socialization. *American Sociological Reviews*, **50**, 530–46.

Zinberg, N. E. (1979). Nonaddictive opiate use. In *Handbook on drug abuse* (ed. R. L. Dupont, A. Goldstein, and J. O'Donnell), pp. 303–14. National Institute on drug abuse, Washington.

6

The image of 'progressive disease'

MARY ALISON DURAND

INTRODUCTION

A chapter entitled 'The Image of "Progressive Disease" ' must by virtue of the title contain some reference to the term 'disease'. This term has many uses and meanings in contemporary medicine and psychiatry and has been applied to alcoholism in a variety of ways throughout the past three centuries. The value of labels cannot be negated: they determine, in part, our perceptions of and subsequent responses to objects, events, and processes. The application of the term 'disease' to alcoholism, for instance, has led clinicians and researchers alike to focus on particular aspects of alcoholism and has, in part, determined the nature of popular treatment strategies.

In considering the term 'disease', however, we must not overlook the adjective 'progressive' as it is surely the nature of the beast, progressive or otherwise, rather than the label that is applied to it which is of primary importance. Increasing our understanding of possible pathways of progression and mechanisms of change in alcoholism is crucial in theoretical, clinical, therapeutic, and preventive terms. The most appropriate framework in which to place the study of progression and change in alcoholism must undoubtedly be a biopsychosocial one. Contemporary conceptions of alcoholism approximate this approach to some extent. However, there exists a need for a greater systematic investigation of intrapersonal, psychological processes, such as attributional beliefs and motivation, as mechanisms of progression and change in alcoholism.

The focus of this chapter will, therefore, be the role of psychological variables, and in particular motivation, as factors in progression and change in alcoholism. First, however, it seems appropriate to look briefly at the various conceptions of alcoholism which have prevailed at one time or another during the last three centuries, and at the potential power of labels, in particular the disease label, when applied to alcoholism.

CONCEPTIONS OF ALCOHOLISM

Edwards (1992) has unpicked the threads of the moral, disease, dependence, and problem models of earlier waves of scientific interest in alcoholism in order to trace the development and emergence of the bi-axial concept of alcoholism. I shall attempt here simply to sketch out his view of developments in recent centuries and refer you to his review for greater detail.

Edwards argues that until the eighteenth century people were concerned primarily with the problems caused by drunkenness, and attributed these problems to man's sinful nature. Through the observations of individuals like Rush and Trotter during this century, however, came the view of drunkenness as the product of habit or disease. Setting their model of drunkenness in the framework of a modern path analysis, Edwards suggests that Rush and Trotter viewed alcohol as being inherently addicting and addiction as a disease of the will which could lead to a variety of problems. He argues that instead of being viewed as the originators of the disease concept, Rush and Trotter should in fact be described as 'the progenitors of a psychological view of dependence'.

The nineteenth century, he maintains, witnessed the addition of many useful observations to the dependence or habit model. However, the end of the century brought with it the birth of a strong disease concept of alcoholism. The lesion concept of disease was fashionable at this time (Kendell 1975) and it is unsurprising, therefore, that alcoholism was conceived of as the product of an underlying constitutional or nervous disorder. Treatment became the issue of the day. This period also witnessed the rise of the Temperance Movement whose concerns included public health issues and the problems caused by alcoholism. However, Edwards notes that these divergent views of alcoholism did not lead to conflict as proponents of the disease model were often in favour of temperance while the Temperance Movement gradually changed its conception of alcoholism.

This century has seen two major developments in scientific opinion concerning the nature of alcoholism. The first of these was a new formulation of the disease concept of alcoholism by E. M. Jellinek, who proposed that alcoholism is a chronic disorder, to which several factors, including a constitutional vunerability factor, contribute. Jellinek proposed that there are five types of alcoholism, but only some of these—the gamma and delta forms, and possibly the omega form—are true diseases of addiction. These forms involve loss of control or the inability to abstain from drinking. The individual who suffers from the disease form of alcoholism has a biological sensitivity to alcohol. Jellinek recognized that non-addictive forms of alcoholism could be extremely damaging in their own right because of the problematic consequences of heavy drinking. The hallmark of the true disease of alcoholism, however, is addiction.

The disease model was challenged by the WHO report in 1977 (Edwards *et al.* 1977) which instead of describing alcoholism as a categorical disease described it in terms of the dimensions of alcohol-related disabilities and dependence. The focus of research and treatment was thus shifted away from disease (Edwards 1992). Alcohol related disabilities, or impairments in the functioning of the individual on physical, social, and mental levels, were recognized as concerns in their own right: it was posited that they could exist without dependence and that their presence was not a necessary indication that the individual was destined to become dependent. The dependence dimension was described under the title of the 'Alcohol Dependence Syndrome' as a condition, rather than a categorical disease, which could exist in varying degrees of severity and was framed in terms of learned behaviour. Edwards suggests several reasons for this change in paradigm which include the type of scientific research being undertaken in the 1970s and the demands of international policy makers for a uniform conception of alcoholism.

Alcoholism is, therefore, currently perceived either in terms of a disease, or as a condition involving a group of related phenomena existing in varying degrees of severity and with a variable prognosis.

THE POWER OF THE DISEASE LABEL

The labels which we use to describe phenomena undoubtedly influence our perceptions of those phenomena. The power of labels can perhaps be best exemplified by some of the work of social psychologists on an element of attribution theory. The bias towards making dispositional rather than situational attributions about the causes of an individual's behaviour has become known as the 'fundamental attribution error' (Ross 1977). This error is operationalized, for example, under conditions whereby an individual has been labelled a 'deviant'. Thereafter any behaviours exhibited by this person are automatically attributed to his 'deviance'. Were a 'non-deviant' individual to exhibit identical behaviours, due account would be taken by observers of the possible role of situational factors in determining his actions.

The application of the disease label to alcoholism similarly influences our subsequent conceptual understanding and empirical approach to the study of the phenomenon. However, the definition of the term 'disease' is in itself problematic. The late 1960s and the 1970s saw several attempts to produce definitions of the term 'disease' which would accord with contemporary philosophy and practice within the disciplines of medicine and psychiatry (for example Scadding 1967; Kraupl-Taylor 1971; Kendell 1975). Each attempt employed different criteria for defining the term. To a large extent definitions of disease are culturally or socially determined. Indeed, Kendell (1975) has argued that the difficulty in defining the term lies in the very fact that the criteria employed have varied in different places at different points in time. In terms of conceptions of alcoholism, Edwards (1977, 1992) has acknowledged that whether or not the dependence syndrome is to be labelled 'disease' will depend, in part, on social, cultural, and political dictates. One might speculate, however, that when people apply the disease label to alcoholism, although they may be willing to acknowledge the role of non-biological factors and the existence of non-biological consequences, they are essentially speaking of a biologically based entity. Three examples will suffice to illustrate the influence of the disease label when applied to alcoholism.

First, the definition of alcoholism as a disease by Jellinek has led proponents of the disease model to concentrate on a search for biological bases of alcoholism and has generated a range of systematic investigations of potential neurological, endocrinological, metabolic, and genetic factors. Blum and Payne (1991), in their book, *Alcohol and the addictive brain*, suggest that the animal and human experiments which have taken place as a result of Jellinek's conceptualization of alcoholism as a disease have not only provided new understanding of disease processes, but have also afforded new medical insights which in turn have strengthened methods of treatment.

Second, the labelling of alcoholism as a disease has led to specific treatment strategies. For example, the disease concept of alcoholism has flourished under the auspices of Alcoholics Anonymous. Alcoholics Anomymous is probably the largest provider of help for people with drinking problems: it claims to have more than 1 500 000 members worldwide and to hold more than 73 000 meetings weekly (General Service Office 1987). A fundamental belief of this fellowship is that alcoholism is a progressive disease, probably taking the form of an allergy to alcohol, which once contracted cannot be cured. The best one can hope for is to arrest the condition (Robinson 1979). Alcoholics are, therefore, called upon to admit to their powerlessness over alcohol, to give their lives up to a power greater than themselves, and to abstain completely from alcoholic beverages. While none of the reviews which have been conducted within the past 20 years (for example Bebbington 1976; Miller and Hester 1986; Emrick 1987, 1989) have found overwhelming evidence to suggest that AA is more effective than other forms of treatment or than no treatment at all, there is some evidence to suggest that individuals who attend AA subsequent to medical treatment do better in terms of drinking outcome than do those who do not attend (for example Hoffman *et al.* 1983). Emrick (1987), on the basis of an extensive literature review, concluded that about 40–50 per cent of those who become active members of AA have several years of abstinence while involved with the programme, and 60–80 per cent show some improvement while involved with the organization.

The third example of the power of the disease label concerns its policy implications. By labelling alcoholism a disease, one implicitly enshrines the right of the alcoholic to medical treatment in the way that individuals suffering from other medical conditions are entitled to such treatment. Furthermore, if alcoholism is seen as a disease then governments are obliged to provide funding for both treatment and research programmes. Thus the image of alcoholism as a disease has been promoted by various interest groups and has become the focus of public health and prevention campaigns, particularly in the USA, in recent decades. As a result numerous surveys have been conducted to gauge the level of acceptance of the concept in the general population and among treatment personnel (for example Caetano 1987, 1989).

BEYOND THE LABEL: PROGRESSION AND CHANGE

While labels are obviously important, the danger is that in considering alcoholism as a progressive disease, we may become so preoccupied with the debate surrounding the usefulness, or otherwise, of the term 'disease' that we ignore the adjective 'progressive'. This is a descriptor which has provoked an enormous amount of debate and interest among those interested in alcoholism treatment and research, regardless of whether they have chosen to think of alcoholism in terms of disease or dependence. It is a concern with the potentially progressive nature of the beast that links former and current conceptions of alcoholism. Rush and Trotter, in the eighteenth century, spoke of disease and habit, suggesting a gradual process, taking place over a period of time. Jellinek (1952) delineated phases in the progressive disease of alcoholism. Edwards (1977, 1992) similarly described mechanisms of behavioural and physiological progression within the framework of the Alcohol Dependence Syndrome. What is common to all perspectives is the desire to describe and explain the mechanisms underlying the process by which some individuals become, over a period of time, dependent or diseased drinkers.

There is, however, a fundamental distinction between talking about progression in terms of alcoholism and progression in terms of disorders such as cancer. Progression in alcoholism is evident only while the individual chooses to drink: a negative outcome is, therefore, not necessarily indicated for the alcoholic in the way that it is for the victim of an incurable form of cancer. As Vaillant and Milofsky (1982) have put it:

over the short term alcohol dependence often resembles a remitting but progressive illness like multiple sclerosis; over the long term, amongst those who survive, alcoholism often resembles a self-limiting illness.

A wealth of clinical evidence points to the fact that positive as well as negative changes can occur in the course of an individual's detrimental involvement with alcohol. The results of both population and clinical studies (for example Vaillant and Milofsky 1982; Hasin *et al.* 1990) suggest that people move in and out of problematic drinking and that people do sometimes stop drinking. The old adage 'once a drunk, always a drunk' does not seem to hold. However, the individual who has become dependent or diseased, even if he is currently abstinent, differs from other drinkers. Relapse has been shown to lead to rapid reinstatement, leading to speculation, for instance, about the existence of addiction memories.

The study of mechanisms of progression and change in alcoholism and of the factors which influence the course and speed of progression and change is important in many ways. We need to know more about the natural history of alcoholism for both theoretical and practical reasons. It is only by understanding more clearly the processes and factors involved that we begin to provide more effective treatment strategies, for instance. The best approach to the study of mechanisms of progression and change in alcoholism must undoubtedly be a biopsychosocial one. The three elements—biological, psychological, and social —are integral to the functioning of the individual in his day to day existence and each has its role to play in his involvement with alcoholism. Concentration on one dimension alone will never allow us to build a complete picture of potential mechanisms of change in alcoholism.

To some extent contemporary perspectives do approximate a biopsychosocial approach to the study of the processes involved in alcoholism. As already noted, a legacy of Jellinek's disease formulation has been the systematic search for potential biological bases of alcoholism.

Edwards (1977) defined the Alcohol Dependence Syndrome as a psychophysiological condition, stating that the compartmentalization of psychological and physiological dependence would be detrimental to the understanding of the syndrome. The dependence model has encouraged the systematic study of the role of psychological and physiological processes in alcoholism within a learning theory framework. Thus, for example, the work that was originally begun by Wikler in the 1940s on classically conditioned responses to alcohol and alcohol-related cues has become the focus of much experimental interest in recent years, particularly in terms of the development of models of relapse (Drummond *et al.* 1990) and of the formulation of treatment techniques such as cue exposure. Similarly, behavioural variables, such as actual drinking behaviour, have become the focus of systematic study. The recognition of alcohol-related disabilities as concerns in their own right has in turn led to the study of these variables as precursors or concomitants of change. The relationships between alcohol-related disabilities, dependence, and consumption have also begun to receive research attention (for example Drummond 1991).

Within the emerging biopsychosocial framework, however, the role of intrapersonal, subjective, psychological variables and factors in alcoholism is not receiving enough theoretical or empirical consideration. There is no denying the importance of the search for biological bases of alcoholism or the importance of establishing models of progression and relapse based on learning theory principles. These endeavours, however, must not be allowed to blind us to the fact that the individual functions as a psychological as well as a biological, behavioural, and social being. His involvement with alcohol has meaning for him at a psychological level. Tapping this meaning in a scientific and systematic fashion can only add to our understanding of mechanisms of progression and change in alcoholism. In advocating more widespread investigation of subjective variables and processes the intention is not to try to resurrect the so-called moral model of alcoholism. It is rather to emphasize that when we speak of the 'alcoholic' or the 'problem drinker' we must remember that we are in fact talking about an individual who experiences motivations and emotions in relation to his use of alcohol and who holds attributional beliefs about responsibility and control, concerning its use. Similarly, he experiences life events that are either related to or independent of his drinking behaviour which may so impinge upon his psychological functioning that they cause him to change that drinking behaviour and so alter the course of his involvement with alcohol (Saunders and Allsop 1985). Indeed, one might speculate that subjective factors may prove not only to be valuable explanatory constructs in the description of progression and change in alcoholism: they may also prove to be the variables which are most amenable to influence in the psychotherapeutic setting.

Much valuable work has already been conducted, investigating variables such as locus of control (for example Canton *et al*. 1988) and attributional beliefs about the causes of change in drinking behaviour (Edwards *et al*. 1987, 1992) but much remains to be done. There are of course methodological and conceptual problems to be overcome in the study of such subjective variables; relevant theoretical formulations and principles need to be employed, definitions of terms need to be clarified, and standardized methods of investigation and measurement established. However, the exploration of processes of change in alcoholism based on psychological theories and principles should not be allowed to lag behind other areas of investigation. A brief review of some work that has been and is being done on motivation as a potentially important explanatory construct of progression and change in alcoholism should suffice as a statement of both the conceptual and practical insights that are to gained from the systematic study of such variables.

MOTIVATION AND ALCOHOLISM

Motivation is a variable commonly spoken about in relation to alcoholism, and in particular in relation to treatment for alcoholism. While there is some evidence to suggest that clinicians tend to support a disease concept of alcoholism (for example Ferneau and Paine 1972; Orcutt *et al*. 1980) and while Blum *et al*. (1989) have speculated that clinicians and researchers have a tendency, from a policy perspective, to be more positively disposed to concepts of disease which are free from attributions of personal responsibility, there is also a wealth of evidence to suggest that attributes of the individual such as commitment, willpower, and motivation are perceived by clinicians as crucial determinants of treatment outcome (for example Sterne and Pittman 1965; Musil 1982; Miller 1985). Indeed, Sterne and Pittman (1965) suggested that alcoholism probably provokes more concern about a patient's motivation to recover than any other 'illness'. Motivation receives some further consideration in Robin Davidson's chapter in this book.

In the treatment setting, motivation has often been perceived as a static variable or trait displayed by the alcoholic: the stronger his motivation, the better the treatment outcome. Traditionally, motivation has been consensually defined by clinicians in terms of the alcoholic's willingness to accept the clinician's definition of the problem, his level of distress, and his compliance with the treatment regimen (Miller 1985).

Davies (1979), however, refuted the static view of motivation, while Miller (1985), in a review of the literature on motivation for treatment, with particular reference to alcoholism, delineated the negative consequences of employing a trait model of motivation and proposed instead that motivation should be viewed as a dynamic product of patient, therapist and situational characteristics.

Factors involved in motivation for treatment have been described as falling into two categories: those which lead the individual to recognize that he has a problem and needs to seek help and those involved in sustaining the desire to stop drinking, once that desire has been aroused (Aharan *et al.* 1967). Much of the existing literature on motivation tends to focus on the assessment and description of motivation in the alcoholic patient from the point of treatment entry onwards. Far less attention has been paid to the processes that bring problem drinkers to treatment in the first place (Jordan and Oei 1989). Much of the work which does exist on help seeking tends to focus on the description of the sociodemographic characteristics of those attending treatment centres (for example Allan 1989). However, Hingson *et al.* (1982), in a large population study in Boston, found that while consumption levels or loss of control over drinking were factors which forced people to acknowledge that they had a problem, social problems and undesirable personal states were the factors which motivated them to seek treatment. Similar findings have been presented by Thom (1987) and Stokes (1977).

Motivation should not be perceived as a variable which is relevant only to helpseeking and treatment outcome. Rather, it is a variable which can be postulated to have a role to play at every stage of an individual's involvement with alcohol, from social drinking to dependence, abstinence, and relapse. Furthermore, motivation is not something which operates in a vacuum: it is influenced by external events and processes as much as by internal states. It may be closely related to beliefs about control and responsibility (Deci 1975), and to expectations and affect (Cox and Klinger 1988).

One can pose a number of basic questions about the potential role of motivation in relation to progression and change in alcoholism. What is it, for instance, that motivates people to drink in the first place? What drives some people to drink in a manner which differs from that of their peers and causes them to persist even when the consequences become aversive? What forces individuals to recognize that their drinking has become problematic and motivates them to do something about it? How do motivational factors influence abstinence and relapse?

In attempting to answer these questions and to thereby formulate explanatory motivational models of alcohol use, clinicians and researchers are becoming increasingly interested in the underlying dimensions and structure of motivation. In accordance with trends in contemporary psychological theories of motivation, drive and drive reduction are no longer the only explanatory constructs used to describe motivated behaviour. Rather, as Cox and Klinger (1988) note, current approaches to motivation are couched in terms such as incentives, goals, and current concerns and involve related variables such as values and affect.

Cox and Klinger (1988) suggest that current theories of motivation have much to offer our understanding of alcoholism and the effectiveness of various treatment strategies. They have formulated a motivational model of alcohol use based on the theoretical construct of incentive motivation. They suggest that the pursuit of incentives forms an integral part of the individual's psychological functioning. An incentive is defined as any object or event which has the capacity to produce affective change or the expectation of affective change in the individual. Cox and Klinger postulate that alcohol use may bring about affective change in the individual either directly through its chemical or expected chemical effects or indirectly through its effects on other incentives in his life. Their model of alcohol use

depicts people as deciding to drink or not to drink on the basis of whether the positive affective consequences they expect to derive from drinking outweigh those they expect to derive from not drinking.

They suggest that the non-chemical incentives in individuals' lives constitute a primary determinant of their motivation to use alcohol, in that people

are motivated to bring about affective changes through the use of alcohol to the extent that they do not have satisfying positive incentives to pursue and to the extent that their lives are burdened by negative incentives that they are not making satisfactory progress towards removing.

Cox and Klinger suggest that the decision to drink or not reflects a combination of rational, or decision making, and emotional processes, but that these are largely 'non conscious and automatized'. They list several so-called historical factors which impinge on the individual's decision to drink: these include the individual's biochemical reactivity to alcohol; his personality characteristics; sociocultural and environmental influences; past reinforcement from alcohol; and, the individual's conditioned reaction to alcohol. The situation in which the individual finds himself at any given time and the nature of the incentives which are currently providing him with positive or negative affective experiences are also cited as factors which influence the decision to drink.

This model is conceptually valuable because it places the individual's involvement with alcohol within the framework of the myriad of other influences in his life. Its practical value lies in the fact that, as Cox and Klinger suggest, it can explain the failure of reinforcement strategies which focus only on drinking behaviour; it can help account for relapse; and it is consistent with the clinical observation that abstinence is associated with non-chemical incentives in the individual's life (for example the findings of Valliant and Milofsky 1982).

Recently, I and some colleagues at the Addiction Research Unit have been attempting to explore the underlying structure of incentives for seeking treatment in alcoholic patients, using the theoretical model of intrinsic motivation proposed by Deci (1975). Briefly, Deci describes intrinsic motivation as consisting of one class of actions which are performed for their own worth rather than for reward and of a second class of actions designed to narrow the gap between the individual's perceived and ideal self-image. Extrinsic motivation, on the other hand, involves actions which are little valued for themselves, but performed contingent upon a reward. An intrinsic incentive for seeking treatment might, for example, be the fact that the individual's current self-image as a down-and-out alcoholic is incongruent with his ideal self-image and seeking help may represent part of the process of changing that current negative self-image. An example of an extrinsic incentive might be the threatened loss of a job, with participation in treatment perceived as a means of preventing that loss. One can speculate that there are many intrinsic and extrinsic incentives for seeking treatment, and that treatment requirements and outcomes may be related to the types of incentives which motivate individuals to seek help in the first place.

The aims of this exploratory study include testing the validity of employing the theoretical framework of intrinsic motivation in assessing the structure of alcoholic patients' motivational incentives for seeking treatment, and exploring possible relationships between incentives for seeking treatment and variables such as dependence, alcohol-related problems, attributional beliefs, and sociodemographic and treatment history characteristics. Although this work is at an early developmental stage, the type of theoretical and practical questions that it raises are important. What, for instance, is the nature of the relationship, if any, between severity of dependence and incentives for seeking treatment? Similarly, is there a relationship between alcohol-related problems and incentives for help-seeking? Is treatment outcome related to initial incentives for seeking treatment? One could speculate, for example, that the intrinsically motivated person might remain abstinent longer post-treatment than the extrinsically motivated one, on the grounds that the former may see abstinence as part of an ongoing process of improving self-image, while the latter, having received his 'reward' (for example saving his job) finds that his motivation to remain abstinent soon flags.

If this is the case, should clinicians be trying to foster intrinsic motivation in alcoholic patients? Questions of this sort can only be answered with the help of longitudinal studies.

Motivation, therefore, seems to represent a potentially interesting explanatory variable in the search for a greater understanding of the mechanisms of progression and change in alcoholism. In order to realize the potential of this variable, however, we must provide clearer definitions of the term, generate standardized forms of measurement and observational analysis, and most importantly, we must recognize that motivation is a dynamic variable, which operates not in a vacuum, but in conjunction with biological, behavioural, social, and other psychological processes.

CONCLUSIONS

While the labels which we apply to phenomena are fundamentally important in that they influence to some extent how we perceive and react to these phenomena, it is necessary in the case of alcoholism to go beyond the debate over the use of the disease label and to focus instead on the nature of progression and change in alcoholism. It is only through the careful examination and analysis of change in the natural history of alcoholism that we can begin to understand the phenomenon. The most appropriate framework in which to place the study of mechanisms of change must surely be a biopsychosocial one, in which changes in the individual's involvement with alcoholism can be examined at all levels of his being and functioning. Current conceptions of alcoholism have fostered and encouraged the examination of processes of change on many levels—the behavioural, the social, and the physiological. The challenge to the future is to increase our knowledge of psychological processes as mechanisms of change in alcoholism.

REFERENCES

Aharan, C. H., Ogilvie, M. A., and Partington, M. A. (1967). Clinical indications of motivation in alcoholic patients. *Quarterly Journal of Studies on Alcohol*, **28**, 486–92.

Allan, C. (1989). Characteristics and help-seeking patterns of attenders at a community-based voluntary agency and an alcohol and drug-treatment unit. *British Journal of Addiction*, **84**, 73–80.

Bebbington, P. E. (1976). The efficacy of Alcoholics Anonymous: the elusiveness of hard data. *British Journal of Psychiatry*, **128**, 572–80.

Blum, K. and Payne, J. (1991). *Alcohol and the addictive brain: new hope for alcoholics from biogenetic research*. Maxwell MacMillan International, New York.

Blum, T. C., Roman, P. M., and Bennett, N. (1989). Public images of alcoholism: data from a Georgia survey. *Journal of Studies on Alcohol*, **50**, 5–14.

Caetano, R. (1987). Public opinions about alcoholism and its treatment. *Journal of Studies on Alcohol*, **48**, 153–60.

Caetano, R. (1989). Concepts of alcoholism among Whites, Blacks and Hispanics in the United States. *Journal of Studies on Alcohol*, **50**, 580–2.

Canton, G., Giannini, L., Magni, G., Bertinaria, A., Cibin, M., and Gallinberti, L. (1988). Locus of control, life events and treatment outcome in alcohol dependent patients. *Acta Psychiatrica Scandinavica*, **78**, 18–23.

Cox, W. M. and Klinger, E. (1988). A motivational model of alcohol use. *Journal of Abnormal Psychology*, **97**, 168–80.

Davies, P. (1979). Motivation, responsibility and sickness in the psychiatric treatment of alcoholism. *British Journal of Psychiatry*, **134**, 449–58.

Deci, E. L. (1975). *Intrinsic motivation*. Plenum Press. New York.

Drummond, D. C. (1991). Alcohol-related problems and public health. MD thesis, University of Glasgow, UK.

Drummond, D. C., Cooper, T., and Glautier, S. (1990). Conditioned learning in alcohol dependence: implications for cue exposure treatment. *British Journal of Addiction*, **85**, 725–43.

Edwards, G. (1977). The Alcohol Dependence Syndrome: usefulness of an idea. In *Alcoholism: new knowledge and new responses* (ed. G. Edwards and M. Grant), pp. 136–56. Croom Helm, London.

Edwards, G. (1992). Problems and dependence: the history of two dimensions. In *The nature of alcohol- and drug-related problems* (ed. M. Lader, G. Edwards, and D. C. Drummond), pp. 1–14. Society for the Study of Addiction, Monograph 2. Oxford University Press, Oxford.

Edwards, G., Gross, M. M., Keller, M., Moser, J., and Room, R. (1977). *Alcohol-related disabilities*. WHO Offset Publication, No. 32. World Health Organization, Geneva.

Edwards, G., Brown, D., Duckitt, A., Oppenheimer, E., Sheehan, M., and Taylor, C. (1987). Outcomes of alcoholism: the structure of patient attributions as to what causes change. *British Journal of Addiction*, **82**, 533–45.

Edwards, G., Oppenheimer, E., and Taylor, T. (1992). Hearing the noise in the system. Exploration of textual analysis as a method of studying change in drinking behaviour. *British Journal of Addiction*, **87**, 73–81.

Emrick, C. D. (1987). Alcoholics Anonymous: affiliation processes and effectiveness as treatment. *Alcoholism: Clinical and Experimental Research*, **11**, 416–23.

Emrick, C. D. (1989). Alcoholics Anomymous: membership characteristics and effectiveness as treatment. In *Recent developments in alcoholism*, Vol. 7 (ed. M. Galanter), pp. 37–53. Plenum Press, New York.

Ferneau, E. and Paine, H. J. (1972). Attitudes regarding alcoholism: the volunteer alcoholism clinic counsellor. *British Journal of Addiction*, **67**, 235–8.

General Service Office of Alcoholics Anonymous (1987). *World AA Directory*. AA World Service, New York.

Hasin, D., Grant, B., and Endicott, J. (1990). The natural history of alcohol abuse: implications for definitions of alcohol use disorders. *American Journal of Psychiatry*, **147**, 1537–41.

Hingson, R., Mangione, T., Myers, A., and Scotch, N. (1982). Seeking help for alcohol problems: a study in the Boston Metropolitan area. *Journal of Studies on Alcohol*, **43**, 273–88.

Hoffman, N. G., Harrison, P. A., and Belille, C. A. (1983). Alcoholics Anonymous after treatment: attendance and abstinence. *International Journal of the Addictions*, **18**, 311–18.

Jellinek, E. M. (1952). Phases of Addiction. *Quarterly Journal of Studies on Alcohol*, **13**, 673–84.

Jordan, C. M. and Oei, T. P. S. (1989). Help-seeking behaviour in problem drinkers. *British Journal of Addiction*, **84**, 979–88.

Kendell, R. (1975). The concept of disease and its implications for psychiatry. *British Journal of Psychiatry*, **127**, 305–15.

Kraupl-Taylor, F. (1971). Part 1: A logical analysis of the medico-psychological concept of disease. *Psychological Medicine*, **1**, 356–64.

Miller, W. R. (1985). Motivation for treatment: a review with special emphasis on alcoholism. *Psychological Bulletin*, **98**, 84–107.

Miller, W. R. and Hester, R. K. (1986). The effectiveness of alcoholism treatment. In *Treating addictive behaviours; processes of change* (ed. W. R. Miller and N. Heather), pp. 121–74. Plenum Press, New York.

Musil, J. V. (1982). A comparison of the views of Czechoslovakian and American psychologists and psychiatrists toward alcoholism. *Journal of Studies on Alcohol*, **43**, 252–60.

Orcutt, J. D., Cairl, R. E., and Miller, E. T. (1980). Professional and public conceptions of alcoholism. *Journal of Studies on Alcohol*, **41**, 652–661.

Robinson (1979) *Talking out of alcoholism: the self-help process of Alcoholics Anonymous*. Croom Helm, London.

Ross, L. (1977). The intuitive psychologist and his shortcomings: distortions in the attribution process. In *Advances in experimental social psychology*, Vol. 10 (ed. L. Berkowitz), pp. 174–214. Academic Press, New York.

Saunders, B. and Allsop, S. (1985). Giving up addictions. In *New developments in clinical psychology* (ed. F. N. Watts), pp. 203–20. John Wiley in association with the British Psychological Society, London.

Scadding, J. G. (1967). Diagnosis: the clinician and the computer. *Lancet*, **ii**, 877–82.

Sterne, M. W. and Pittman, D. J. (1965). The concept of motivation: a source of institutional and professional blockage in the treatment of alcoholics. *Quarterly Journal of Studies on Alcohol*, **26**, 41–57.

Stokes, E. J. (1977). Alcoholic women in treatment: factors associated with patterns of help-seeking. Doctoral dissertation, Brandeis University, USA.

Thom, B. (1987). Sex differences in help-seeking for alcohol problems. 2. Entry into treatment. *British Journal of Addiction*, **82**, 989–97.

Vaillant, G. E. and Milofsky (1982). Natural history of male alcoholism. IV Paths to recovery. *Archives of General Psychiatry*, **39**, 127–33.

7

Understanding smoking relapse: predisposing factors, precipitating factors, and a combined model

STEPHEN SUTTON

INTRODUCTION

This book is about change. Sadly and all too evidently, one very possible type of change is the event of relapse.

Relapse is the modal outcome in smoking cessation programmes and self-initiated attempts to quit. Most smokers who quit in the short term go back to smoking within a few months. It is important to try to learn more about the process of relapse, its antecedents and sequelae, so that intervention programmes can be improved and the basis of the smoking habit can be better understood.

Two main research strategies have been used to study smoking relapse. The first investigates smokers' reasons and attributions for relapse and the situational antecedents and concomitants of relapse episodes. This will be referred to as the *situational* approach and the term *precipitating* factors used. Not surprisingly, studies employing this approach are usually retrospective. The second main approach investigates predictors of relapse with the aim of identifying factors that may predispose smokers to relapse. Research of this type has typically employed prospective designs in which relapse/maintenance is predicted from characteristics assessed at baseline. This will be termed the *predispositional* approach or as the study of *predisposing* factors. While this approach addresses the question 'Who relapses?', the situational approach deals with the 'When?', 'Where?', and 'Why then?' of particular relapse episodes.

Using this distinction, this chapter aims to give a highly selective review of recent ideas and research in the area of smoking relapse. For more detailed and comprehensive—though less topical—reviews of the literature, see Sutton (1989) and Niaura *et al.* (1988). To date, the two research strategies I have identified have been pursued separately. The last part of the chapter will show how the two appoaches can be combined by outlining a simple framework incorporating both predisposing and precipitating factors. The notion of 'motivated relapse' will also be briefly discussed. Although, the focus throughout is on smoking relapse, the ideas and research findings discussed are applicable, in principle, to the problem of understanding relapse in the other addictive behaviours. Indeed, many authors have stressed the commonalities among the addictive behaviours in respect to relapse (for example Brownell *et al.* 1986). Before commencing the review proper, it is useful by way of background to discuss briefly the issue of how to define relapse and to present some data on relapse rates.

DEFINITION

Relapse means going back to smoking after a period of voluntary abstinence. Definitions of relapse have differed with respect to:

1. The minimum period of abstinence that qualifies a smoker to be eligible for relapse.

2. What counts as 'going back to smoking'.

Taking the second aspect first, it is useful to split the process of relapse into two stages and to distinguish, as many others have, between the first 'lapse' or 'slip' (defined as the first puff or the first cigarette following a period of abstinence) and subsequent smoking behaviour, which might involve regaining of abstinence, further lapses, or resumption of smoking at the original consumption level (a 'full-blown' relapse).

The minimum qualifying period of abstinence has ranged from 24 hours to one year. There is an advantage in using a relatively short period in that it enables one to incorporate time off cigarettes as an independent or moderating variable in the analysis, so that it is possible to examine, for example, the question of whether the factors that predict early relapse differ from those that predict late relapse.

Many studies that purport to investigate relapse do not in fact do so. In order to be considered directly relevant to relapse, the sample for analysis should consist only of smokers who have stopped smoking for some minimum period of time; those who have not stopped and those who stopped but have already relapsed should be excluded from the analysis so that relapse is not confounded with cessation. For example, in a treatment study in which outcome at six months is predicted from various measures assessed at the end of treatment, the relevant sample might be those abstinent at the end of treatment. This has the additional advantage of controlling for the confounding effects of end-of-treatment smoking status. Unfortunately, many studies do not report analyses based on abstinent subjects only.

Although most studies use a dichotomous outcome (relapsed/maintained abstinence) at a given follow-up point, a few studies have measured the number of days, weeks, or months to first lapse or to resumption of regular smoking (for example Stevens and Hollis 1989). Such data enable the more powerful techniques of survival analysis to be applied (Singer and Willett 1991) in addition to the traditional regression analysis. However, it is difficult and costly to obtain sufficiently detailed and precise data on time to relapse.

Most studies treat relapse as the endpoint of a linear succession of states (smoking → abstinence → smoking, or in the case of the 'successes', smoking → abstinence). What happens to the subject after they have relapsed is usually not the focus of interest. An alternative approach is to view this as one relatively brief episode in an ongoing stream of behavioural change. Adopting a wider time-window than is employed in the typical treatment study would allow the possibility of studying the movement between spells of abstinence and spells of smoking. To my knowledge, only one study to date has investigated this approach (Swan and Denk 1987).

RELAPSE RATES

In the early 1970s, Hunt and his colleagues published relapse curves obtained by averaging the results of a large number of treatment studies. Fig. 7.1 is taken from Hunt and Bespalec (1974) and shows the cumulative survival curves for two sets of studies; the 1971 curve is based on 87 studies, the 1973 curve on 89 studies. Note that the 1973 curve shows an increase in the percentage of abstainers between the first and second follow-up points instead of the expected monotonic decrease. This anomaly is presumably a result of combining disparate studies using varying follow-up periods, treatments, subject samples, and definitions of outcome. Some cautionary comments on the interpretation of relapse curves can be found in Litman *et al.* (1979) and Sutton (1979).

Of those subjects abstinent at the end of treatment, the proportions still abstinent at the 9–18-month point are in the range of 20 to 35

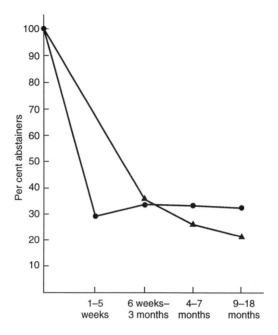

FIG. 7.1 Cumulative survival curves for two sets of treatment studies (from Hunt and Bespalec 1974, showing relapse rate over time. ●, 1973; ▲, 1971.

per cent. The data indicate that most smokers relapse, and most relapses occur, within the first three months.

The best data on long-term relapse rates in a treatment or intervention setting come from the Multiple Risk Factor Intervention Trial (MRFIT), a six-year clinical trial of heart disease prevention through risk factor modification conducted in the United States. Since I refer to this study again later, I will briefly describe the trial here.

Men aged 35–57 at high risk for heart disease were randomly assigned to Special Intervention (SI) and Usual Care (UC) groups. Cigarette smokers in the SI group attended 10 weekly group sessions incorporating both health education and behaviour modification components and then entered either a maintenance or an extended intervention programme which involved regular attendance (at least every four months) at the MRFIT centres. Fig. 7.2 shows the survival curve for the SI group based on data from Hughes *et al.* (1981). There were 3596 men who were cigarette smokers at first screen and who attended the 48-month follow-up visit. Of these, 1676 (46.6 per cent) had stopped by the 4-month follow-up (which marked the end of the intensive intervention

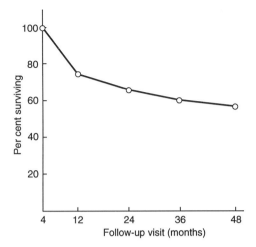

FIG. 7.2 Cumulative survival curve for the Special Intervention (SI) group in the Multiple Risk Factor Intervention Trial (MRFIT) based on data from Table 7 in Hughes *et al.* (1981).

stage). This group is represented by the first point on the curve (100%). At 48 months, 56.2 per cent were still abstinent. It should be noted that these data are based on subjects' self-reports and that those who switched to a pipe or cigars were counted as successes. Although most relapses occurred in the first half of the period, significant relapse nevertheless took place after the 16-month follow-up (that is, approximately one year from the end of the intensive intervention); a third of those who relapsed between four months and 48 months did so after the 16 month point.

PRECIPITATING FACTORS: THE SITUATIONAL APPROACH

The situational approach involves contacting smokers after they have lapsed or experienced a relapse crisis and asking them to describe the situation in terms of such factors as the location, whether other smokers were present, whether they were consuming food or alcohol at the time or immediately before, their mood state, how they obtained the cigarette, and so on. Of the several coding schemes that have been used in this field, the most popular has been that devised by Shiffman (1982). I know of six studies that have used his coding scheme or a variation on it. The study characteristics and results are summarized in Table 7.1.

TABLE 7.1 Studies of lapse situations that have used Shiffman's (1982) coding scheme: *(From Sutton 1992)*

Variable	Study					
	1	2	3	4	5	6
Sample characteristics						
Sample size (number of lapsers)	70	69	176	186	92	216
Age	—	39.8	36.7	42[a]	31.4	35[a] (median)
Percentage female	66.6[a]	60.9	56.2	53.4[a]	56.5	60.6[a]
Baseline cigarette consumption	34.5[a]	28.3	23.4	24.5[a]	27.3	25.7[a]
Years of previous smoking	19.9[a]	21.7	19.5	22.9[a]	13.5	—
Median number of days abstinent	9.7[a]	57	56.0	—	—	—
Mean number of days abstinent	36.5[a]	82.7	—	—	57.8	—
Minimum number of days abstinent	2	1	7	<1	—	1
Characteristics of lapse situations (percentages)						
Site						
Home	45.7	53	35	33.3[a]	26.4	37
Work	20.0	23	16	26.1[a]	11.3	30
Other	34.3	24	43	40.6[a]	62.3	33
Smokers present	44.9	50	56	43.3[a]	58.5	53
Consumption						
Any	59.3[a]	52	50	—	68.5	30[b]
Alcohol	29.4	21	24	19.7[a,b]	47.2	18[b]

TABLE 7.1 (continued)

Variable	Study					
	1	2	3	4	5	6
Characteristics of lapse situations (percentages) (continued)						
Affect						
Positive	28.8[a]	17	31	—	23.8	32
Negative	71.2[a]	83?	52	—	65.6	56[c]
Neutral	—	—	15	—	—	—
How obtained cigarette						
Asked another for it	—	42	40	—	60.0	—
Bought it	—	39	34	—	23.3	21
Offered it	—	11	4	—	2.2	—
Other	—	8	22?	—	14.5	—
Attributed to problems/crisis/stress	52.0[a]	52	39	55.9[a]	—	40

[a]Based on *total* sample, not lapsers only.
[b]From question about antecedent activities.
[c]Includes 'stressed' as well as the other negative mood states.

Studies: 1. Shiffman (1982)
2. Cummings *et al.* (1985)
3. Baer and Lichtenstein (1988)
4. Bliss *et al.* (1989)
5. Brandon *et al.* (1986, 1990)
6. Borland (1990)

For further details see Sutton (1992), from which source most of the material in this section has been taken.

The clients investigated were all long-term regular smokers. They differed, however, with regard to length of abstinence. This partly reflects an important difference in methodology. Shiffman's (1982) study and that of Borland (1990) recruited subjects via a telephone hotline. This may be a useful way of obtaining information on early relapse crises or lapse episodes, albeit in a highly self-selected sample of smokers. In contrast, the subjects in Studies 2, 3, and 5 were smokers who had stopped smoking while participating in a cessation programme and then lapsed or relapsed during a one- or two-year follow-up period. Subjects in Study 4 were volunteers who were making a serious attempt to quit smoking on their own without formal help; they were interviewed one month after their quit date. In these studies, all those who lapsed were interviewed, thus eliminating the possibility of self-selection bias arising from the use of the hotline methodology.

In spite of these differences and variations in how the questions were asked, some consistent results emerged. Smokers were present in about half the lapse situations. The majority of lapses occurred during or soon after the consumption of alcohol, food, or coffee, and in the majority of cases the informant reported feeling anxious, depressed, angry, or bored at the time of the lapse. A substantial proportion of lapses were attributed to problems, a crisis, or stress. Studies using different coding schemes have also highlighted the frequency with which lapses occur in the presence of a negative mood state (Cummings *et al.* 1980; O'Connell and Martin 1987). When asked how they obtained their cigarette, most subjects said either that they had asked someone else for it or that they had purchased it.

Perhaps of more relevance than the characteristics of lapse situations *per se* are the differences between lapse crises that are survived and those in which the person smokes. Shiffman (1982) identified a number of such correlates. Compared with those who did not smoke, lapsers were significantly more likely to report that other smokers were present, that they had consumed alcohol, and that the crisis took place at sites other than home or work. Negative affect was not related to outcome. The most important predictor of outcome was performance of a coping response. Ex-smokers who reported using either behavioural coping (for example refusing the offer of a cigarette, leaving the situation) or cognitive coping (for example mentally reviewing the benefits of quitting) were much less likely to smoke than those who performed no coping response (28 vs. 58 per cent for behavioural coping; 30 vs. 55 per cent for cognitive coping). Shiffman (1984) showed that the number and to a large extent the type of coping responses was unrelated to survival.

Support for these findings comes from a study of unaided quitters reported by Curry and Marlatt (1985). They suggest that treatment participants should be encouraged to 'think *and* do something' when they encounter a high-risk situation. None of these authors comment on the difficulty of distinguishing between behavioural coping (presumed to be a determinant of outcome)—refusing the offer of a cigarette, for example—and the outcome itself (that is not smoking in that situation).

PROBLEMS WITH THE SITUATIONAL APPROACH

There are obvious problems with such retrospective data. It is difficult to catch people immediately after a relapse crisis or lapse episode when the circumstances are still fresh in their mind. Retrospective descriptions may be unreliable, they are impossible to validate, and they may be subject to self-presentational bias, or to bias due to subsequent events and experiences (for example whether or not a lapse becomes a full-blown relapse).

Data of the kind reviewed above have been interpreted as indicating that some situations (for example negative mood state, presence of other smokers) are associated with a high risk of lapse. The concept of risky or tempting situations appears frequently in the literature. Most of these situations cannot be avoided; it is simply a matter of time before the recent ex-smoker will encounter one of them. On this view, staying off smoking depends on successfully negotiating such high-risk situations by being prepared for them and by employing coping strategies that have been rehearsed beforehand. This, in a nutshell, is the basis of the relapse prevention approach advocated by Marlatt and Gordon (1985) and which is seen as applicable across the range of the addictive behaviours.

It should be noted that the terms 'risky' and 'tempting' carry somewhat different connotations. 'Risky' and 'high risk' imply simply that the probability of lapsing is relatively high in that situation. The term 'tempting', on the other hand, has more specific connotations. In particular, it suggests that there is something about a given situation that makes an ex-smoker think about and desire a cigarette while simultaneously feeling that they should try to resist the urge. Conditioning theories of one kind or another have often been used to explain why some situations are risky or tempting and others are less so. For example, one idea that occurs in the literature on opiate and alcohol dependence is that withdrawal symptoms such as craving and irritability may become classically conditioned to environmental cues and that relapse may be due to conditioned withdrawal (for example Niaura *et al.* 1988; Wikler 1980).

There is a problem with interpreting the data on lapse situations as evidence for the existence of high-risk situations. Although a substantial proportion of lapses take place when people are experiencing negative emotional states, for example, it does not follow that such states are high-risk situations. It may just be that they are very common situations, and that, other things being equal, relapse is more likely in a frequently-experienced situation than in an unusual situation. It is conceivable that negative emotional states are actually relatively low-risk situations. Smokers who are trying to quit may experience numerous episodes of boredom, anger, or depression without lapsing. Thus, the conditional probability of lapsing, given a negative mood state, may be relatively low. The proportion of lapses that occur in negative affective states (that is the kind of data reported above) depends on both the *frequency* with which such states are experienced and the *riskiness* of such situations defined in terms of the conditional probability of lapsing given that state. The point can be illustrated with an extreme example: virtually all lapses take place when people are wearing clothes. Does this mean that wearing clothes is a high-risk situation for smoking and should be avoided in order to maintain abstinence?

This analysis raises the question of the frequency of exposure to different situations among smokers who are trying to quit. We need data on exposure to situations during the period prior to the first lapse. Instead of focusing on those situations in which lapses did occur (the positive instances), we also need to look at those situations in which lapses did not occur (the negative instances). Extending this approach, it would be valuable to try to relate three sets of situations: usual smoking situations; situations encountered when the person tries to quit; and the situations in which the first and subsequent lapses occur.

As a postscript to this section, Saul Shiffman is already addressing this problem of base rates by equipping his experimental subjects with hand-held computers programmed to beep at random time intervals and to prompt the subject to enter ratings of mood and other data. This method of *experiential sampling* may lead to significant advances in our understanding of the situational determinants of relapse.

PREDISPOSING FACTORS

Other studies have employed a different approach to investigating smoking relapse. Baseline information is obtained from a group of recent ex-smokers and they are followed up to find out who maintains abstinence and who relapses. The aim is to identify predictors of outcome which may indicate factors that predispose an individual to relapse. The term 'predisposing' (like the term 'precipitating') implies causal influence and the factors discussed in this section should be regarded as predisposing factors only in a provisional or potential sense.

This approach can be illustrated by the data in a recent paper from the MRFIT group (Hymowitz *et al.* 1991). They identified a sample of almost 1000 men who were initially cigarette smokers, who quit during the first year of the trial, and who reported smoking zero cigarettes/day at the first annual visit, confirmed by salivary thiocyanate levels. They defined a relapsed quitter as a 12-month quitter who at any subsequent annual visit, up to and including six years, reported smoking or whose thiocyanate level exceeded the cut-off or for whom either piece of information was missing. They then tried to predict the dichotomous smoking status variable (relapsed/maintained abstinence) from baseline information obtained before the cessation attempt was made.

The relapse rates at six years were 22.5 per cent in the SI group and 39.8 per cent in the UC group. These are lower than most other reported figures, presumably because of the relatively long qualifying period of initial abstinence, although the authors do not state how long the 12-month quitters had been abstinent from cigarettes. Thus, on the face of it, this study appears to be an investigation of factors associated with late relapse; the predictors of early relapse may be different.

Factors not found to be significantly related to relapse in either group included the following: age; race (black vs. other); marital status (married vs. other); wife smoking status (yes/no); expectation of quitting (yes/no); number of five best friends who smoke; Jenkins Activity Survey score (Type A); and cigarette consumption. The last finding is of particular interest for two reasons. First, cigarette consumption was an important predictor of cessation in this study, suggesting that the predictors of cessation and relapse may differ. Second, it appears discrepant from findings reported in an earlier paper on the MRFIT study (Hughes *et al.* 1981). In that paper, the authors used a 4-month qualifying period and a 48-month follow-up period and found that the relapse rate among heavy smokers was substantially higher than among lighter smokers.

In all but one case, factors that were predictive of relapse were significant in the UC group only. Those subjects with fewer years of education were more likely to relapse. Those who had quit smoking in the past were more likely to relapse (42.3 per cent) than those who had not previously attempted to quit (17.4 per cent). Those who had experienced more life events prior to quitting were more likely to relapse. And, finally, those who drank more (as measured by reported number of alcoholic drinks/week) were more likely to relapse. The relapse rate was 21.1 per cent among those who reported zero drinks/week compared

TABLE 7.2 *Factors found to be predictive of relapse/maintenance in selected recent prospective studies of smoking relapse*

Self-efficacy for recovery of abstinence (Haaga & Stewart 1992)

'Withdrawal symptoms' (Daughton *et al.* 1990)

Negative affect smoking (O'Connell and Shiffman 1988)

Social support (Havassy *et al.* 1991)

Belief that smoking during pregnancy will increase an unborn child's chance of getting sick (Quinn *et al.* 1991)

---

with 56.3 per cent among those who consumed 22 or more drinks per week. This was the only factor that was significantly predictive of relapse in the SI group.

Other factors that have been found to be predictive of relapse in recently published studies are shown in Table 7.2. All these studies were prospective and in all cases the analysis was based on initially abstinent subjects only. This is not a comprehensive list of recent findings or studies. It is included simply to give an idea of the kinds of factors that been investigated.

Although considered here under the heading of predispositional factors, a term which implies a relatively enduring property, the factors listed may differ with respect to stability and malleability. For example, confidence in one's ability to stay off cigarettes is likely to fluctuate during the attempt to quit. Very low levels of self-efficacy (and possibly very high levels) may trigger a lapse. In this sense, self-efficacy can be regarded as a precipitating factor. However, the distinction between predisposing and precipitating factors is not clear-cut: a change in the level of a predisposing factor, particularly a sudden change, may have an effect similar to a transient situational precipitant such as smelling cigarette smoke. Simply on an empirical basis, if a factor measured at baseline is shown consistently to predict relapse then it is appropriate to consider it as a potential predisposing factor. Shiffman (1989) has a very useful discussion of the distinction between predisposing and pre-cipitating factors and a third category which he calls background factors.

A COMBINED MODEL

To summarize, this chapter has reviewed recent work on smoking relapse in terms of two main approaches: a retrospective one focusing on the immediate antecedents of a lapse or slip, and a prospective one in which

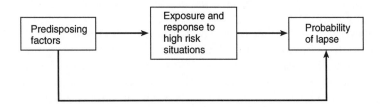

FIG. 7.3 A simple model of lapse combining predisposing and precipitating factors.

lapse or relapse is predicted from baseline characteristics. It seems that if progress is to be made in this field we need to combine these approaches and conduct prospective studies in which both kinds of data are collected. Only one study has investigated both predisposing and precipitating factors in the same subjects (O'Connell and Shiffman 1988). To encourage discussion of a combined approach and to guide future work in this area, the simple, provisional framework shown in Fig. 7.3 is proposed.

The model assumes a defined time period (for example six months) and has three main elements:

1. **Predisposing factors**. These are relatively stable individual differences characterizing recent ex-smokers. The term is defined broadly to include demographic variables, personality, and attitudinal variables, biological factors, and so on.

2. **Exposure and response to high-risk situations**. The label *exposure* refers to the likelihood, frequency and pattern of exposure to high-risk situations in a given time period, as well as the variety of situations encountered. *Response* refers to the cognitive, affective, physiological, and behavioural response to the situation (excluding smoking). The type and characteristics of the situation (for example the number of smokers present) would also fall under this heading. Such characteristics and the individual's response to the situation are potential precipitating factors. They are of course conditional on exposure to a high-risk situation.

3. **The probability of lapsing in the defined time period.**
Stated simply, what the model says is that there are unspecified predisposing factors that influence the likelihood that an individual will encounter particular kinds of situation, the ex-smoker's cognitive, affective,

physiological, and behavioural response to a given situation, and hence the probability of lapsing. To give an example, recent ex-smokers who are relatively heavy drinkers (a predisposing factor) will be more likely to encounter situations in which alcohol is available (a precipitating factor) and will, therefore, be more likely to lapse within a given time period following their quit date than their lighter drinking or teetotal counterparts. Given that they find themself in such a situation, their baseline alcohol consumption and/or other predisposing factors may influence the strength of their desire to smoke and their ability and motivation to use some suitable coping response (for example drinking low-alcohol lager). As a second example, a smoker who is prone to depression (a predisposing factor) will be more likely than other smokers to experience negative affect situations (a precipitating factor) while they are trying to quit and their response to such situations may depend on their depression-proneness and on other predisposing factors.

Of course, particular kinds of smoker may be more likely to lapse in particular kinds of situation. In other words, we might expect to find statistical interactions between personal and situational variables. Thus, the smoker with a drinking problem may not only be more likely to encounter a situation in which alcohol is available but, given that he/she does encounter such a situation, their probability of relapsing may be greater than that of a teetotaller in the same situation.

Fig. 7.3 also shows an arrow going directly from predisposing factors to lapse probability. This is intended to indicate that predisposing factors may have a direct influence on the probability of lapse that is not mediated through exposure to high-risk situations or through the ex-smoker's responses in such situations.

CONCLUSIONS

Relapse is usually seen as an event, as something that happens to the unfortunate smoker who is trying to quit smoking, as a kind of accident or mistake which occurs through carelessness and unpreparedness for dangerous situations. To use an analogy, the recent ex-smoker who suffers a lapse is, on this view, rather like the car driver who has never practised on a skid pan and who, while not concentrating on his driving, hits a patch of black ice and skids off the road. One might, though, favour a rather different view, one that regards relapse not as an event but as an action or decision. The decision may be a 'micro-decision'—to smoke one cigarette—or a 'macro-decision'—to abandon one's attempt to quit. With the possible exception of Marlatt (for example Marlatt and Gordon 1985) who discusses related notions, this idea of 'motivated relapse' has not received a great deal of attention in the literature, but it seems to me to represent an important dimension missing from most current theoretical approaches which emphasize skills and confidence. It can be represented in the model by invoking a predisposing factor called motivation to stay off smoking which would be expected to fluctuate over time and which may influence, and be influenced by, exposure to high-risk situations. If the ex-smoker reaches a point where their motivation to stay off smoking is low, they will be vulnerable to relapse, particularly if their confidence or self-efficacy is also low. Furthermore, an ex-smoker whose motivation is wavering may seek out or engineer a high-risk situation that provides an opportunity to smoke and a sufficient justification for having done so or a way of concealing the transgression. Part of the lapsed ex-smoker's problem, of course, is presentational: how to justify and explain the violation to his/her partner, friends, therapist, and others with an interest in their attempt to quit. For further discussion of decision-making approaches applied to cessation and relapse in the addictive behaviours, the reader is referred to Sutton (1987) and Saunders and Allsop (1987).

REFERENCES

Baer, J. S. and Lichtenstein, E. (1988). Classification and prediction of smoking relapse episodes: An exploration of individual differences. *Journal of Consulting and Clinical Psychology*, **56**, 846–52.

Bliss, R. E., Garvey, A. J., Heinold, J. W., and Hitchcock, J. L. (1989). The influence of situation and coping on relapse crisis outcomes after smoking cessation. *Journal of Consulting and Clinical Psychology*, **57**, 443–9.

Borland, R. (1990). Slip-ups and relapse in attempts to quit smoking. *Addictive Behaviors*, **15**, 235–45.

Brandon, T. H., Tiffany, S. T., and Baker, T. B. (1986). The process of smoking relapse. In *Relapse and recovery in drug abuse* (ed. F. M. Tims and C. G. Leukefeld), pp. 104–17, National Institute on Drug Abuse Research Monograph 72. Department of Health and Human Services, Rockville, Maryland.

Brandon, T. H., Tiffany, S. T., Obremski, K. M., and Baker, T. B. (1990). Postcessation cigarette use: The process of relapse. *Addictive Behaviors*, **15**, 105–14.

Brownell, K. D., Marlatt, G. A., Lichtenstein, E., and Wilson. G. T. (1986). Understanding and preventing relapse. *American Psychologist*, **41**, 765–82.

Cummings, C., Gordon, J. R., and Marlatt, G. A. (1980). Relapse: Prevention and prediction. In *The addictive behaviors* (ed. W. R. Miller), pp. 291–321. Pergamon, New York.

Cummings, K. M., Jaén, C. R., and Giovino, G. (1985). Circumstances surrounding relapse in a group of recent ex-smokers. *Preventive Medicine*, **14**, 195–202.

Curry, S. and Marlatt, G. A. (1985). Unaided quitters' strategies for coping with temptations to smoke. In *Coping and substance use* (ed. S. Shiffman and T. A. Wills), pp. 243–65. Academic Press, New York.

Daughton, D. M., Roberts, D., Patil, K. D., and Rennard, S. I. (1990). Smoking cessation in the workplace: Evaluation of relapse factors. *Preventive Medicine*, **19**, 227–30.

Haaga, D. A. F. and Stewart, B. L. (1992). Self-efficacy for recovery from a lapse after smoking cessation. *Journal of Consulting and Clinical Psychology*, **60**, 24–8.

Havassy, B. E., Hall, S. M., and Wasserman, D. A. (1991). Social support and relapse: Commonalities among alcoholics, opiate users, and cigarette smokers. *Addictive Behaviors*, **16**, 235–46.

Hughes, G. H., Hymowitz, N., Ockene, J. K., Simon, N., and Vogt, T. M. (1981). The Multiple Risk Factor Intervention Trial (MRFIT). V. Intervention on smoking. *Preventive Medicine*, **10**, 476–500.

Hunt, W. A. and Bespalec, D. A. (1974). An evaluation of current methods of modifying smoking behavior. *Journal of Clinical Psychology*, **30**, 431–8.

Hymowitz, N., Sexton, M., Ockene, J., and Grandits, M. S. (1991). Baseline factors associated with smoking cessation and relapse. *Preventive Medicine*, **20**, 590–601.

Litman, G. K., Eiser, J. R., and Taylor, C. (1979). Dependence, relapse and extinction: A theoretical critique and a behavioral examination. *Journal of Clinical Psychology*, **35**, 192–9.

Marlatt, G. A. and Gordon, J. R. (1985). *Relapse prevention: Maintenance strategies in the treatment of addictive behaviors*. Guilford Press, New York.

Niaura, R. S., Rohsenow, D. J., Binkoff, J. A., Monti, P. M., Pedraza, M., and Abrams, D. B. (1988). Relevance of cue reactivity to understanding alcohol and smoking relapse. *Journal of Abnormal Psychology*, **97**, 133–52.

O'Connell, K. A. and Martin, E. J. (1987). Highly tempting situations associated with abstinence, temporary lapse, and relapse among participants in smoking cessation programs. *Journal of Consulting and Clinical Psychology*, **55**, 367–71.

O'Connell, K. A. and Shiffman, S. (1988). Negative affect smoking and smoking relapse. *Journal of Substance Abuse*, **1**, 25–33.

Quinn, V. P., Mullen, P. D., and Ershoff, D. H. (1991). Women who stop smoking spontaneously prior to prenatal care and predictors of relapse before delivery. *Addictive Behaviors*, **16**, 29–40.

Saunders, B. and Allsop, S. (1987). Relapse: A psychological perspective. *British Journal of Addiction*, **82**, 417–29.

Shiffman, S. (1982). Relapse following smoking cessation: A situational analysis. *Journal of Consulting and Clinical Psychology*, **50**, 71–86.

Shiffman, S. (1984). Coping with temptations to smoke. *Journal of Consulting and Clinical Psychology*, **52**, 261–7.

Shiffman, S. (1989). Conceptual issues in the study of relapse. In *Relapse and addictive behaviour* (ed. M. R. Gossop), pp. 149–79. Routledge, London.

Singer, J. D. and Willett, J. B. (1991). Modeling the days of our lives: Using survival analysis when designing and analyzing longitudinal studies of the duration and timing of events. *Psychological Bulletin*, **110**, 268–90.

Stevens. V. J. and Hollis, J. F. (1989). Preventing smoking relapse, using an individually tailored skills-training technique. *Journal of Consulting and Clinical Psychology*, **57**, 420–4.

Sutton, S. R. (1979). Interpreting relapse curves. *Journal of Consulting and Clinical Psychology*, **47**, 96–8.

Sutton, S. R. (1987). Social-psychological approaches to understanding addictive behaviours. *British Journal of Addiction*, **82**, 355–70.

Sutton, S. R. (1989). Relapse following smoking cessation: A critical review of current theory and research. In *Relapse and addictive behaviour* (ed. M. R. Gossop), pp. 41–72. Routledge, London.

Sutton, S. R. (1992). Are 'risky' situations really risky? Review and critique of the situational approach to smoking relapse. *Journal of Smoking-Related Disorders*, **3**, 79–84.

Swan, G. E. and Denk, C. E. (1987). Dynamic models for the maintenance of smoking cessation: Event history analysis of late relapse. *Journal of Behavioral Medicine*, **10**, 527–54.

Wikler, A. (1980). *Opioid dependence: Mechanisms and treatment*. Plenum, New York.

Part III.

Bridging the personal and environmental
explanations of change

8

Environmental influences which promote or impede change in substance behaviour

HARALD K.-H. KLINGEMANN

INTRODUCTION

A discussion of the relative importance of environmental determinants of change in substance behaviour must span a wide conceptual and empirical range. Such change may refer to the onset, the relative increase, the relative decrease, or the complete cessation of the use of various psychotropic substances or of associated problem-behaviour. The change may be linear or include feedback structures in circular models, and may be temporary or permanent. Whether the structure and complexity of such models depend upon the specific substance or are the same for all substances (integrated model of change) is another question for research. The interaction of physiological, psychological, and environmental independent variables must be accounted for before the net effect of environmental variables on the change process, and the ultimate changes, can be assessed.

Within this general framework this chapter presents a review of studies on change in different forms of addictive behaviour, with a focus on environmental variables as determinants of such change, highlights their specific importance and points to the needs of future research. Examples are included from Switzerland, with its unique alcohol legislation and the very high rate of illicit drug use and drug problems.

The evaluation of treatment effects and the support of change in **treated populations** are topics of *relapse studies* discussed in the first section. However, relatively few substance users seek treatment. Also, besides other frequent methodological shortcomings, treatment outcome studies in particular exclude many facets of social function and rarely control for post-treatment environmental variables. Hence, one can hardly take isolated results from such studies at face value.

The chapter then reviews the **natural history of untreated populations**, drawing upon recent examples from heroin, alcohol, and tobacco studies. It focuses on the role of social conditions, particularly social support, in the framework of cognitive *coping models* for various addictive disorders.

Spontaneous remission studies already provide a broader view than analysis of treatment outcome. However, this type of research is still in its infancy and has been criticized for, *inter alia*, using small convenience samples and lacking control groups. The next section draws on general population studies to describe the environmental correlates of substance behaviour. Both longitudinal and cross-sectional studies are discussed under the aspect of *life-events* and stressful life conditions, such as status changes related to ageing, family formation, and employment, as potential determinants of substance use across the life course.

The notion of 'environmental influences' also encompasses the sociocultural milieu as a determinant of individual change. Human development is also linked to social change across the life course. To distinguish between period/time effects, cohort/generation effects, and individual age is a basic requirement in studies of social dynamics (for example Mayer and Huinink 1990). Cross-cultural factors also come into play.

Conditions of change for a 20-year-old drug user of the hippie generation in the 1960s are different from those for a 20-year-old drug user in 1992; female alcoholics did not have specific treatment facilities in Switzerland in the 1960s, 15 years later they did; living in times of a new sobriety, in some countries, changes the environmental contingencies of would-be quitters; while Scandinavian schoolchildren are likely to have readier access to alcohol in the unrestricted EU market of the future than they had 10 years ago.

Surprisingly, studies in the addiction field hardly ever address the relation between aspects of individual, group, and societal change. This is quite a methodological challenge; there is little empirical evidence about links between the aggregate and the individual level. The next section outlines *changes in treatment systems* since World War II, drawing upon the first European Summary of Drug Abuse (ESDA) and the International Study of the Development of Alcohol Treatment Systems (ISDATS) to discuss the *climate of consumption*, the factors that affect the average consumption of licit and illicit drugs, which in turn, at least indirectly, influences the motivation of problem users for change: changing lifestyles, acculturation processes, the role of mass media in the diffusion of norms, and aspects of the *availability* of psychotropic substances.

Some of the discussion will, to a degree, cross-cut with other contributions to this book, particularly the chapter by Reginald Smart. We believe that these different perspectives are complementary and we have not, therefore, tried to avoid all overlap.

THE RELATIVE IMPORTANCE OF INTERPERSONAL ASPECTS OF CHANGE, BY STUDY/SAMPLE TYPE

Monitoring treatment results: social determinants of relapse and maintenance among treated populations

Follow-up studies of clinical samples have often been motivated by therapeutic interests in achieving a lasting treatment impact, for example by broadening or intensifying programmes (for example Foote and Erfurt 1991, on aftercare in Employee Assistance Programmes). Another recurrent theme of such studies has been the question whether the return from problem consumption to normal consumption is possible in the long run. Both themes tend to ignore the intermediate social, physiological, and psychological processes that lead to changes in the outcome variables. Much more instructive for our understanding of individual maintenance is, therefore, the question: under what conditions do the effects of treatment not persist and patients relapse?

The work of Marlatt and Gordon (1980, 1985) exemplifies this approach and is of particular interest because it compares different substances and attempts to depict the relapse process. Their classification system for relapse episodes may serve as a useful frame of reference for the issues here in question. They distinguish between intrapersonal events or reactions to non-personal environmental factors and interpersonal events. The latter category includes direct and indirect social pressure and coping with interpersonal conflict. In a preliminary study of chronic alcoholics they showed that 'the majority of patients began drinking again in the presence of powerful interpersonal forces, thus highlighting the salience of social factors as determinants of relapse' (Marlatt and Gordon 1980). More precisely, circumstances preceding the consumption of the first drink are characterized by frustration in personal relations or social situations. This finding is supported by a follow-up assessment of the circumstances associated with first use, carried out 90 days after the completion of a treatment programme among a larger sample ($n = 137$) of alcohol, heroin, and tobacco users: 42 per cent of all relapses were related primarily to interpersonal factors in 47 per cent of drug addicts, 43 per cent of smokers, and 39 per cent of alcoholics. Moreover, direct social pressure affected mostly alcoholics and heroin addicts, and indirect social pressure mostly smokers (negative models in numerous daily situations) (Marlatt and Gordon 1980). However, taken together, these results underline rather the commonalities of risk situations across the addictions, which became apparent when comparing relapse rates over time (see also the review by Brownell *et al.* 1986, including also obesity). The cognitive-behavioural model of the relapse process presented by Brownell *et al.* includes plausible assumptions about the interaction of interpersonal and intrapersonal variables: abstinence violation can lead to the definition of lapses as relapses, increase helplessness and undermine effective coping behaviour in interpersonal conflict (Marlatt and Gordon 1980; Brownell *et al.* 1986). The cross-cultural replication study by Sandahl (1984) substantiated these findings also for a longer follow-up of treated alcoholics in Sweden: the distribution of relapse situations in the Stockholm study is similar to that in the Seattle study, interpersonal categories accounting for 50 per cent of them (Sandahl 1984). Again, the *importance of social/psychological interactive effects* is emphasized: 'Patients who do not readily adjust to other persons' opinions tend to relapse in interpersonal conflicts and patients who are more impulsive cannot resist social pressure to drink' (Sandahl 1984).

The only observed cultural difference is the private location of the first drink in Sweden (56 per cent at home) and the public setting in the United States (63 per cent in a bar). This reflects the tighter social control of consumption in Sweden. Sandahl also notes that the greater access in Sweden seemingly does not speed up the relapse process and concludes: 'There seems to be a certain amount of universality regarding risk situations between the American and Swedish drinking culture' (Sandahl 1984). It is remarkable that this study speculates on the cultural context effect, but, as we shall see later, period/historical effects (such as the reduction of per capita consumption) are hard to pin down.

In their later review, 'Understanding and preventing relapse', Brownell *et al.* (1986) differentiate the assumption that the risk of relapse is determined by an interaction of psychological, situational, and physiological factors, by referring to various *stage models* of the change process:

Physiological factors may promote lapse and may increase the likelihood of relapse. The environmental and social factors can provide the setting, stimuli and encouragement from others to lapse. As the choice point for the lapse approaches, coping skills can prevent the lapse. Whether the lapse recurs and ends in relapse probably results from a complex interaction of these factors (Brownell *et al.* 1986).

However, *the relevance of cognitive-change variables* characterizing the basic stages: 'motivation and commitment', 'initial behaviour change', and 'maintenance', has been questioned as well as the nature of these interactive effects.

Baar and O'Connor, for example, observe on the basis of a number of (alcohol) case studies that relapse frequently follows a period of success and low anxiety. Therefore, they assume that unconscious and psychotic rather than neurotic processes are at work (Baar and O'Connor 1985). Similar observations have been made about quitters from smoking:

The frequent experience of relapse in **positive** (author's emphasis) moods suggests ... that low level reasoning is due to a lack of mental energy under emotional stress, since stress, whether positive or negative, tends to create excessive demands on the monitoring of mental processes (Sjöberg 1983).

The seven months follow-up of Lando *et al.* to detect effects of a self-help kit for quitting smoking yielded an unexpected result, which also seems to support this line of thought: 'The use of a number of preparation strategies was associated with unsuccessful outcome... the only exception was for use of supportive others' (Lando *et al.* 1991).

One shortcoming of many treatment outcome studies, including those mentioned above, is their very limited time-frame. Do studies with a longer follow-up period confirm the importance of environmental/social factors?

The latest Swiss follow-up study, conducted in 1988, included all male alcoholics treated between 1975 and 1984 in the country's largest alcohol clinic. First, the variability of post-treatment behaviour proved to be considerable, emphasizing the need to expand the time-frame of such studies. The assumption of a 'safe point' after one year of abstinence (Emrick 1975) is only partially supported. The abstinence rate of 48 per cent after the first year kept dropping smoothly to 33 per cent at the end of the third year and to 26 per cent beyond that time (Spinatsch and Chilvers 1991). The social integration before treatment admission (for example employment status, previous sentences) and during the follow-up period (for example living with somebody) determined, to a large extent, the drinking status at the time of interview (Spinatsch Chilvers 1991). More specifically, the difficulties of reintegration immediately after treatment, such as finding a job or an apartment and being exposed to the stigma of a former alcoholic (problems with the authorities), seem to be minor stressors compared with the frequent negative life-events, which seem to have an important potential for relapse: 60 per cent of the subjects experienced the death of a close one, a separation/divorce, an accident or an illness (Spinatsch and Chilvers 1991).

Despite the extended time-frame, the results of this and other studies with a similar design concerning other substances (see the nine-year follow-up of pathological gambling by Blaszczynski *et al*. 1991) can by no means be generalized. Most minimal ground rules for studies on the natural history of clinic treatment are not met: a follow-up period of at least 5–15 years; outcome assessment at multiple different times; prospective studies of admission variables; the inclusion of multiple facets of social function; controlling post-treatment environmental variables; and minimal attrition (Vaillant 1983).

An exception is the eight-year follow-up (1972–1980) of a clinic sample of 110 alcoholics (five reassessments), which was part of the classic study of Vaillant (1983) on the natural history of alcoholism. With regard to environmental factors for change, he presents two basic findings. First, there is an association between the alcoholism and social adjustment (for example employment and marital status) at outcome: 'as a group, the chronic alcoholics were psychosocial cripples and the stable remissions were employed and were living in gratifying social environments' (Vaillant 1983); and second, patients' *social stability* at the time of seeking treatment is important to sustained abstinence (Vaillant 1983).

These results confirm previous findings, as well as those from the Swiss study mentioned above:

Over the short term, social stability is an important predictor of alcoholism outcome. Premorbid marital status, employment, residential stability, first-admission status and the absence of previous drunk arrests all significantly predicted who would become a stable remission by 1979 (Vaillant 1983).

Over the very long term, however, social stability proved not to be such an important predictor of alcoholism outcome, as the comparison with the other samples (the 40-year follow-up of the College sample and Core city sample) showed (Vaillant 1983).

This draws attention to the basic limitations of studies of treatment outcome and the crucial role of 'natural healing forces', and the need for research into 'spontaneous' remission from problem substance use— that is, remission without treatment.

Giving up the deviant career: environmental aspects of spontaneous recovery

Treatment populations represent only a very small sample of the total problem group, and these populations are further biased by varying institutional procedures of patient selection, the over-representation of lower-class male clients, involuntary treatment, and severity of the problem. It cannot be assumed that recovery rates and the reasons for recovery are comparable in treated and untreated samples.

Three literature reviews represent a first baseline for the discussion in this area: Smart (1975/76) on research on natural recovery of alcoholics until 1975; Waldorf and Biernacki (1979) on the incidence literature on heroin addiction until 1978; and Stall and Biernacki (1986) on recovery from smoking and food addiction without professional help. A major conclusion of the first two reviews was that natural recovery *is* not rare and might come close to recovery rates via treatment, but that longitudinal survey designs fail to uncover the underlying reasons and processes of spontaneous remission. Smart (1975/76) therefore concluded at the time that future studies 'should focus on concomitant changes in social stability but also informal "treatment" by friends, relatives and Alcoholics Anonymous'; and Waldorf and Biernacki (1979) made a similar point about heroin studies: 'Future research... must be undertaken to ...learn what are the actual processes of recovery for both treated and untreated addicts—what initiated the attempt to recover, how the individuals cope and what kind of interpersonal, familial and community support are utilized'.

Consequently, subsequent research in this area has, more and more, been focused on **the nature of the process of natural recovery**. It has used smaller samples and active case-finding methods, testing *inter alia the hypothesis of the importance of social support* as the counterpart of interpersonal conflict. The follow-up study by Kendell and Staton (1966) is an early example of changing research perspectives. Their study showed that demographic standard variables such as social class, sex, and age had little relevance; but it supported the assumption that social stability at the workplace and in the family, as well as the development of satisfying personal relationships, constituted favourable conditions for spontaneous remission. Saunders and Kershaw (1979) came to similar conclusions in their analysis of retrospective interviews with former problem-drinkers: 'The mechanisms behind this process appear to involve the establishment of new, or improved significant relationships, the termination of alcohol-related employment and other changes in life circumstances'.

Although these studies emphasized a more dynamic view of change in individual behaviour than did classic longitudinal surveys, later and more qualitative research, based mainly on the life-history approach, has provided a 'close up' of the individual development of natural recoveries. The following short review focuses upon the evidence from this research during the early 1980s on environmental factors promoting individual change.

The study of Tuchfeld (1981) is based on a non-representative small sample ($n = 51$) of subjects who reported that they had resolved their drinking problems without any formal treatment and that they had sustained abstinence for at least one year. The findings suggested a stage of problem recognition, disengagement, interim changes in alcohol-related behaviour, and sustained change in alcohol-related behaviour. In the first phase, strong aversion was revealed to any form of professional intervention and to being labelled. In the second phase, perceived reasons of change were health problems, the confrontation with negative role models, and extraordinary crisis-situations. Permanently maintaining tentative changes in behaviour finally depended on the individual's ability to cognitively support such a commitment ('justifying rhetoric'), but especially on the effectiveness of informal social control exercised by family and friends, and a background of favourable professional and financial conditions (Tuchfeld 1981). The study of Stall (1983) takes the same direction. In the early stages of natural recovery, Stall differentiates between situation- and crisis-induced drinking as well as problem drinking as a result of social isolation. As to maintenance, Stall's findings are congruent with those reviewed in the Tuchfeld study: during the disengagement and stabilization phases it appears that support received from significant others is of paramount importance for the course of 'spontaneous' remission (see also Brady 1993).

Finally, studies on 'spontaneous' remission from illicit drugs tend to support those findings. In the work of Waldorf and Biernacki (1981) as well as Waldorf (1983), the role of informal support systems is also stressed, particularly in connection with identity transformation through contact with alternative-religious and other ideological groups. Graeven and Graeven (1983) point out that, in accordance with the labelling perspective, spontaneous remissions often occurred among those individuals who had relatively strong family support and little contact with the criminal justice system. In addition to geographical change as a coping strategy, Blackwell (1983) reports on effective self-medication during the attempt to stop using a substance (for example hot baths or taking alcohol) and, particularly, reliance upon the informal help of family and friends.

On the whole, all these findings point to a certain agreement on the stages in spontaneous remission from alcohol and drugs and the importance of interpersonal factors.

The review by Stall and Biernacki (1986) of findings related to alcohol, illicit drugs, smoking cessation, and eating disorders broadens this perspective and tries to integrate them into a comprehensive stage model. Comparisons of studies of these various addictive disorders show that similar social and psychological conditions for successful natural recovery are at work: changes in relationships with significant others are paramount both in initiating and in sustaining spontaneous remission;

other important factors include becoming conscious of the health and financial consequences of substance abuse, personal processes of change, reference to significant experiences, the ability to manage craving, and the external reinforcement of conforming behaviours (Stall and Biernacki 1986). In view of these findings, from an interactionist perspective it can generally be concluded that 'the central process which underlies spontaneous remission is the successful public renegotiation and acceptance of the user's new, nonstigmatized identity' (Stall and Biernacki 1986).

The authors propose *a three-stage model*. The first stage deals with building up motivation in the 'user trying to cure himself', the second with the public negotiation of a new, non-stigmatized identity, and the third with stabilizing the higher conformity achieved in the sense of abstinence or controlled consumption.

According to Stall and Biernacki, what triggers the user's decision in the first stage to change behaviour is primarily financial and health problems, but also having to cope with social sanctions and difficulties with significant others. In the second stage, in which a redefinition of identity is not only based on major lifestyle changes but also burdened by cravings, active social support is of crucial importance. Access to such supporting networks is assumed to be a relevant stabilizing factor during the third stage, in addition to the positive feedback resulting from having put an end to the substance abuse career.

Brownell *et al.* (1986), who also stress the commonalities across the addictions, complete the picture by proposing specific methods for the prevention of lapse and relapse corresponding to the described stages of their natural history.

Although this type of research is still in its infancy, most recent studies on the autoremission phenomenon have avoided a number of methodological shortcomings of the previous work and assume some kind of a stage model. The four-year follow-up Canadian study of a sample of alcohol remitters, by Sobell *et al.* (1992), included a control group of non-resolved, non-treated alcohol abusers; in Switzerland, a longitudinal comparative study of the natural history of alcohol and heroin use is under way (Klingemann 1991); and Tucker and Gladsjo (1993) conceptualize individual help-seeking on a continuum (combinations of 'no treatment'—'AA attendance'—'formal treatment'), investigating its influence on the current drinking status of an American sample. More specifically, attention has also shifted towards a more detailed analysis of behavioural strategies used by self-quitters (for example Oei and Hallam, 1991, 1992*a*).

Do the findings of these more elaborate studies contradict or support previous research; and how important are environmental circumstances that promote or impede change, according to these studies?

The analysis by Tucker and Gladsjo (1993) of the determinants of help-seeking and long-term recovery status shows that situational factors are more influential than stable characteristics of drinkers and standard diagnostic criteria. Treatment entry was associated with greater alcohol-related psychosocial problems (not necessarily higher consumption), especially in interpersonal relationships, and the authors conclude:

The functional value of treatment entry for individual clients within the context of environmental circumstances surrounding entry implies that it may have less to do with client interest in stopping drinking than with resolving problems in relationships with significant others.

As to the untreated resolved subjects who had relatively high dependency levels prior to the solution, the findings showed an interaction effect between decreasing alcohol-related physical problems and on greater vocational stability as well as less overall life disruption. On the basis of this functional approach, the lack of gender-specific differences between the groups is no surprise to the authors:

Rather than focusing on sex as a static predictor variable, future research should focus on how gender roles may contribute to ... environmental variables that motivate or deter help seeking and problem resolution.

The authors conclude that both treatment-seeking and recovery status are connected with the functional consequences of consumption.

Complementary to these findings, first results of the Sobell *et al.* (1992) study show that 57 per cent of their recovered subjects had previously included such consequences as costs and benefits of consumption in a cognitive or appraisal process. At the same time, no significant differences were found between the groups (including the 'nonresolved, nontreated' control group) for the full life-event scale. This supports the view that the functional meaning of such events probably cannot be captured by counting discrete events without considering their sequential order across the life course and situational-event clusters. The additional hypothesis of Sobell *et al.* that resolution-related events would differ by age cohort addresses such a context effect. The younger age cohort reported more maintenance factors and more reasons not to seek treatment than the older groups, probably because of different lifestyles and a less stable environment. However, for all three age cohorts, spousal support was the factor most frequently named by subjects as helping them maintain their recovery (Sobell *et al.* 1991). Other forms of social support, such as friends and family, were very important as well. Intrapersonal and non-personal, notably 'self-control/ willpower change' (64 per cent) and physical health change (48 per cent), seem to complement the positive change effect (Sobell *et al.* 1993,

Table 2 therein), much as in the Tucker and Gladsjo study mentioned above.

However, the widely held assumption of the important role of social support for natural recovery has been differentiated by the latest study in Switzerland, which included measures of perceived and received social support in stressful life-events. Both heroin and alcohol remitters, but especially the former, perceived the potential of available post-resolution help to be higher, and indicated having received support when under stress much more frequently than before recovery (number of friends and resource persons) (Klingemann 1992*a*). While this refined measurement confirms previous findings, the analysis of coping and implementation strategies shows a quite different picture. Before the resolution, three-quarters of quitters felt rather isolated and tended to adopt individualistic strategies for coping with craving. The relative importance of individual bias in the perception of help and the deliberate retreat from social relationships in this vulnerable phase may serve as a tentative explanation. Again, the motivation to change is to a large extent determined by **positive** changes (75 per cent) in personal relationships (Klingemann 1991). Substance-specific factors also come into play: the increased stress for illicit-drug users seems to distort the perception of available help. Also, even after their successful recovery heroin quitters are exposed to more social stigma than the alcohol remitters (Klingemann 1992*a*).

The Swiss study found life philosophies/world views to be a mediating factor between social stress or social resources and maintenance. Compared with samples of the general population, heroin and alcohol quitters are much more inner-directed and convinced that they are responsible for their life and can change it. However, the higher stigma experienced by the heroin, compared with the alcohol, quitters, seems to be buffered by an identity change characterized by post-materialist values (Klingemann 1990, 1992*a*): frequently they become helpers themselves, including the possibility of the professionalization of a former deviant identity (Brown 1991).

Examples from recent research on unaided successful quitting by smokers complete the picture. To begin with, the studies of both Oei and Hallam (1991) and Lando *et al.* (1991) emphasize the cognitive build-up of motivation as a preparatory strategy for quitting. Practically all subjects thought of reasons to quit. However, a closer look reveals contradictory findings about the role of social support. Lando *et al.* identify 'reliance on supportive others' as the only factor discriminating successful quitters not specifically seeking treatment from unsuccessful cases (Lando *et al.* 1991), but Oei and Hallam's sample of untreated ex-smokers reported mainly individual health problems as a reason for quitting smoking; to please or 'benefit someone' was not important (Oei and Hallam 1991). Behavioural coping strategies for resisting smoking are manifold, vary in their perceived usefulness, and differ from professional perspectives in quit-smoking programmes. More than 50 per cent of the subjects in Oei and Hallam's sample found all of the eight reported behavioural strategies very useful*. More precisely: '...aversive and positive reinforcement strategies might have greater appeal to would-be quitters than physiological strategies and/or graded habituation' (Oei and Hallam 1991). Again, the study of Lando *et al.* (1991) found very few differences between the strategies of successful and unsuccessful quitters: while both groups think frequently about benefits, successful quitters are motivated less than unsuccessful quitters by considerations of the negative effects of smoking or by the reactions of others to smoking.

These results, which may be flawed by methodological shortcomings or specific circumstances, are difficult to interpret. The study of Lando *et al.* took place in the context of a larger programme, on community prevention; the social support effect during the preparation phase, therefore, might be partially due to this very condition. To what extent Oei and Hallam's study used open-ended questions is not clear; possible interpersonal implications of their strategy categories which might show up in the qualitative material collected cannot be deduced from the Tables presented. Also, Oei and Hallam do not discuss interaction effects —for example of positive reinforcement and the subjective importance of social reactions. Nevertheless, it can be assumed that the importance of *social support as an environmental condition of the different stages of natural recovery varies with substance*. One might speculate about the more general reasons for this (see also pp. 146–53): Distancing techniques, for example 'to stay away from other consumers', become progressively more difficult to implement as the substance changes from cigarettes to alcohol to illicit drugs. Manipulating access, that is 'to make the substance difficult to get', varies similarly: in Switzerland milk is more difficult to buy than beer, which can be purchased almost round the clock, and cigarette machines are everywhere, for everybody. Whether substance abusers can involve supportive others in reaching their goals, which is our main interest in this context, will depend upon the stigma attached to the addictive behaviour and the associated varying helplessness or willingness of others to help when they are confronted with such problems. Recent research has emphasized that relationships involve

---

* How sophisticated and multidimensional everday causal concepts are, compared with scientific thinking, has also been demonstrated with respect to social problems in general (Klingemann 1992c)

benefits and costs and pointed to the salience of upsetting events within a social network (Pagel *et al.* 1987). A clearer empirical distinction between the perception and evaluation of social support, the actually received support, and the structural social integration (Barrera 1986; Klingemann 1988) might clarify the assumed prominent role of social support during the remission stages and possibly reconcile seemingly contradictory findings.

To illustrate this point, Jung (1986) from his study on coping responses of significant others to problem drinkers concludes that:

most ... are concerned about the problem drinker, since about half of them talk to other friends and family about the problem; yet, over one-third seem to feel powerless since they avoid the task of doing something, a form of denial perhaps.

Research on the effects of significant others on change in health behaviour in other areas (for example exercise, salt use, consumption of fat, misuse of prescription medicine) has shown the need to distinguish more carefully different forms of interpersonal support, as overall supportiveness is assumed to be more helpful than other changes in health habits or encouragement (Zimmerman and Connor, 1989). Moreover, different types of primary groups can provide different forms of assistance (Kail and Litwak 1989).

Life events and changing situational factors determining substance use across the life course

The findings presented so far, on the relative importance of environmental influences on change, have been based only on treated populations or convenience samples of untreated subjects. The methodological problems that do not permit the generalization of these results have been listed above. We shall, therefore, turn to a third category of studies, using samples of the general population to describe the concomitants of changes in substance use, in this case alcohol consumption.

The guiding perspective of most of these studies has been the assumption that stressful life situations and life events will lead to increased alcohol consumption. The study of Romelsjö *et al.* (1991) and Temple *et al.* (1991) are prominent examples of the few prospective studies in this category. The longitudinal study of Romelsjö *et al.* was based on a large Californian sample and investigated the relationship between consumption change (1965–1974), stressful life conditions (1965), and life events, such as the death of a loved one (occurring 1966–1973, reported 1974). The results do not support the initial assumption:

Little indication was found that stressful life conditions, life events (losses) and psychosocial factors are importantly associated with change in alcohol consumption ... other factors such as environmental restrictions and pricing seem to be more important in predicting change in consumption in natural populations (Romelsjö *et al.* 1991).

Selected results from the ambitious collaborative alcohol-related longitudinal project, including a cross-cultural meta-analysis of 12 studies, do not support the hypothesis of the effect of stressful life-events. Temple *et al.* (1991) use prospective data and highly sophisticated methods to examine the broader question of the relationship between role changes (marital and employment status) and changes in drinking, and conclude: 'Few of the changes were found to be significantly related to consumption in a statistical sense'.

These longitudinal studies investigate mainly cohort effects, but the relevance of environmental factors may change also as a function of age and life cycles. The passage of juveniles to adult status and the transition from working status to retirement with age are institutionalized changes in the life course and may also be associated with variation in substance behaviour.

As to the *status changes of youths* the basic question is whether behaviour such as deviance in adolescence determines adult behaviour. General factors such as early unemployment or family formation (for example Power and Estaugh 1990*a*), or specific conditions such as subcultural preferences (for example Hagan 1991) and differential primary group associations (for example Orcutt 1987), are among the environmental influences discussed in this area. More specifically, Power and Estaugh (1990*a*) observe that 'changes in drinking were associated with the rate at which young adults formed their partnership and family' and that early unemployment seems to favour heavier drinking in men (Power and Estaugh 1990*b*). On the whole, however, the results are far from conclusive and the direction of the relationships is unclear.

A constant cross-sectional finding is a decrease in heavy drinking among *older age strata* compared with younger cohorts. However, there has been little research on the identification of 'natural factors' favouring decrease in alcohol use with aging (Stall 1986*a*). Brennan and Moos (1991) refer to a stress and coping framework to analyse samples of late-onset drinkers, early-onset drinkers, and non-problem drinkers. The late-onset drinkers tended to live in more benign life contexts, but again, like Romelsjö *et al.* (1991), no evidence was found 'of an association between age-related loss events and the onset of late-life drinking problems'. The in-depth study of Stall (1986*b*), based on a small sample of a 19-year follow-up of a general household survey, focused on respondent-identified reasons for change in alcohol-related behaviour during the second half of the life course. The relative importance of social reasons over psychological/health reasons was equally high for subjects decreasing their alcohol intake (42 vs. 15 per cent) and for those who had increased it (62 vs. 14 per cent). However, most interesting in this context is the:

puzzling aspect of the analysis ... that men who increased use sometimes identified the same factors as explanations for increase as did men who decreased use. Social networks and the experience of retirement were two such variables ... the crucial factor ... is not the experience of certain ... life events, but rather how such events are woven into the aging person's life history.

This conclusion raises the question why life-event research on addiction has shown only limited results so far.

Stall and other life-history researchers (for example Öjesjö 1991) assume that only measurement of the individual configuration of life events, and assessment of the meaning of the circumstances in the individual life course, would resolve the apparent contradiction that in many cases the same variables are associated with increase and decrease (Romelsjö *et al*. 1991). This also touches upon the problem of temporal ordering of life events, which in none of these studies could properly be established. Gorman and Peters' (1990) in-depth study of life events preceding onset of alcohol disorders in a small sample ($n = 23$) of hospital patients illustrates very well the necessity of a precise 'mapplng out' of the events.

Moreover (cf. the discussion on a more valid measurement of social support or social resources), the measurement concepts of stressful life circumstances should also distinguish between undesirable sudden events and long-term strains (Moos and Sindle 1990). Intracategory variability (Dohrenwend *et al*. 1990) and the role of the level of pre-existing chronic stress as a determinant of the experienced stressfulness of specific life events also have to be taken into consideration (Wheaton 1990).

Regardless of these methodological difficulties, a dynamic life-course perspective, relating different life events and situations, provides a useful frame of interpretation, as examples from cross-sectional risk-factor studies show.

Trice and Sonnenstuhl (1990) point out that the reduction of *workplace* risks must not only consider classical intra-organizational risk factors such as work stress, alienation, social control, and occupational subcultures, but also 'build upon naturally occurring social processes of advice giving and receiving'. Clarke *et al*. (1990) emphasize that the impact of workplace factors cannot be generalized but depends upon the general development of drinking patterns across the lifetime: 'Risk factors may contribute to the development and maintenance of drinking styles which lead in the long term to physical disease but do not appear to influence the drinkers who present in the first instance for alcohol treatment' (Clarke *et al*. 1990).

Risk factors for juveniles in the *family* context are another example. The extent to which onset of, or change in, substance use among youth is determined by parental smoking/drinking, etc. models has been discussed in countless studies. Green *et al*. (1991) show that the interaction of gender roles and social class as a context factor leads to important differentiations: parental drinking behaviour was associated positively with young people's drinking only in non-manual classes and among daughters. Needle *et al*. (1986) focus on the role of peer groups and older siblings influencing adolescent drug use and offer an interesting life-course interpretation:

These questions take on greater importance because of the increasing significance of the sibling bond over the life course due to shrinking family size, longer life span, divorce and remarriage, geographical mobility, maternal employment and alternative sources of child care, and various forms of parental insufficiency. Siblings have the potential for being the longest-term relationship ... over the life course.

The intracategory variability of situations and events can finally be illustrated by the Goor *et al*. (1990) observational study of the influence of situational factors on *adolescent* drinking rates in typical group situations. The consideration of overall drinking-situation variables as well as drinking-group and individual variables was more fruitful than a conservative static 'frequency of exposure to leisure type drinking' approach. Similarly, 'zooming in' on drinking occasions shows differences in the perceived appropriateness of drinking by beverage type and social context (Klein and Pittman 1990) Thus, drinking frequency and quantity during a given life stage might also covary with the meaning of a drinking event and the expected reactions of others.

BEYOND THE GROUP PERSPECTIVE—THE EFFECTS OF THE SOCIOCULTURAL ENVIRONMENT ON SUBSTANCE BEHAVIOUR

Changes in treatment

Treatment-seeking is one option, though perhaps not a very important one as spontaneous-remission studies indicate, which the individual can consider as helpful for the resolution or the maintenance phase. The structure of the treatment system, co-determining the client's objective and perceived access, will partially define the relative usefulness of the treatment option. Instead of a cross-sectional analysis of the help-seeking process, the discussion will focus upon the question of how changes in the treatment system can promote or impede change in substance behaviour.

According to the cross-cultural ISDATS study (International Study of the Development of Alcohol Treatment Systems, Klingemann and Takala 1987) important quantitative and qualitative changes have taken place since World War II. While large differences remain in the ways in which different countries regard alcohol and tackle alcohol problems, most of the 16 countries represented in the study (mainly in Europe and North America) have much in common. Most obviously, almost all have seen a large growth in alcoholism treatment. This general increase has been associated with increasing deinstitutionalization, decentralization, and a differentiation of available treatment. Outpatient treatment has become more prominent, treatment responsibilities often have shifted to the community level, and mutual-support groups such as Alcoholics Anonymous have gained a foothold, particularly in the Nordic and anglophone countries, to mention just a few examples (Klingemann *et al.* 1992; Mäkelä 1991).

As regards the treatment field in illicit drug use, the first ESDA report (European Summary on Drug Abuse), based upon reports from 30 countries of the World Health Organization European Region, reveals similar trends. Between 1985 and 1989/90 drug-specific treatment also expanded, according to 16 of the country reports, especially in Southern Europe. Owing to concern about the HIV/AIDS epidemic, the number of low-threshold facilities has been increased in Denmark, Netherlands, Germany, and Switzerland; outpatient treatment is becoming more common and psychiatric treatment is playing a smaller part. Another development of note is an increase in lay help and self-help and in non-governmental activities (Klingemann 1992*b*).

How do these findings relate to change in individual behaviour? What characteristics of treatment systems support or impede change?

The assumption that the general growth of treatment industries and 12-step programmes will improve individual potential for change has already been questioned in discussing research on the natural processes of recovery. In his entertaining and provocative book, *Diseasing of America*, Stanton Peele (1989) expresses the opinion that people quit addictions usually on their own, and goes one step further, outlining the negative effects of the 'therapeutic colonisation of our lives': '... addiction treatment is becoming more pervasive and coercive, and today holds out the possibility of corrupting our society and the self-conceptions of its members'. More specifically, he claims that more treatment for everything and everybody undermines self-efficacy, the feeling that people can control the outcomes in life that matter to them. The disease model leads addicts to interpret relapses as proof that they are powerless in the face of their addictions (Peele 1989). Moreover, on the basis of a literature review by Miller and Hester (1986) Peele assumes: 'Successful treatments ... deal with addicts' interactions with their environments and help them develop beliefs in their self-efficacy' (Peele 1990–91). This argument is not new. Vaillant (1983) concluded that the attention of the therapist should be redirected to the individual's own power of resistance, and that 'we need to study the special role that health-care professionals play in facilitating those (natural healing) processes' (Vaillant 1983).

On qualitative changes in treatment, the data from the ESDA monitoring exercise and the ISDATS study show a differentiated picture. The American experience to which Peele refers can by no means be generalized. Countries vary greatly in the relative weight they accord to such basic concepts as 'cure', 'care', or 'control', reflecting the modes in which societies react to the problems. The concept of alcoholism as a disease has gained some ground, but is still far from being universally regarded as a discrete, irreversible disease (Miller 1986; Klingemann *et al*. 1992). Similar variance is to be found in the *goals of treatment*. More and more, the classic requirement of abstinence as the only acceptable goal of treatment has lost ground. The Swiss case is typical:

Whereas abstinence was a central requirement for appointment between 1950 and 1970, only 19% of the supervisors hired between 1973 and 1983 were required to be abstinent. Most counsellors take alcohol themselves and many institutions have changed their names during the last 10 years, eliminating moral connotations and broadening their institutional goals to include prevention and substance abuse (Klingemann 1984; Klingemann *et al*. 1992). It might be assumed that treatment systems based on social or mixed models offer better conditions for change and give more room for natural healing processes.

Peele's observation that there is more reliance on *coercion* is not supported by other country experiences. On the contrary, voluntary forms of treatment play a greater role in most treatment systems (Klingemann and Takala 1987) and should, according to the theoretical assumptions presented above, increasingly facilitate change in substance behaviour. Especially the ESDA report shows the diversification of treatment programmes and a growing acceptance of low-threshold and maintenance/drug prescription programmes that provide aid for survival and aim at the reduction of individual stress and drug-related problems.

Similarly, *minimal intervention programmes*, such as the use of self-help manuals in Scotland (Heather 1986) and Switzerland (Noschis 1988/89), create favourable conditions for the combined effects of social and professional support. These forms of 'assisted spontaneous recovery' might avoid, to some extent, the negative attitudes to treatment reported in natural recovery studies (Klingemann 1992*a*). Finally, the differentiation of treatment has group-specific effects, often accompanied by increasing privatization. Consequently, support for 'chronic cases' has diminished, because treatment providers try to attract other kinds of clients (Tecklenburg 1986; Klingemann *et al.* 1992). Therefore, changing regulations for the financing of treatment affect directly the individual's possibilities of seeking treatment.

Social change

Treatment systems, however, may not be the most effective agents of change in substance behaviour. For instance, in alcohol research the 'distribution of consumption' theory assumes that the heavy drinking of a minority in a given society is to some extent linked to the accepted norms and behaviour patterns shared by the majority. How exactly, and why, are not very well understood. Skog (1985) hypothesizes that:

flux of direct and indirect influences between individual drinkers in a social network will tend to tie the whole population together. The product of this process can be conceived as a general field of social forces, which influence the drinking behaviour of practically all members of the network... each individual drinker will adjust his drinking according to the mean consumption level in his culture.

How fast the diffusion of consumption norms (for example elements of the drinking culture) proceeds depends, according to Skog, on the nature of social networks and the magnitude of the consumption change on the group members' susceptibility to sociocultural pressure. If one accepts the flexible concept of the 'alcohol dependence syndrome' and a gradual transition from normal to abnormal drinking, then the impact of changes in the general drinking culture is considerable.

Changing lifestyles and cultural transition

Societal norms and values are important conditions for individual opportunities of change and characterize modes of social control. The decline of per capita alcohol consumption in many countries since the early 1980s (Smart 1989) has been explained, at least partially, by the increasing popularity of *healthy lifestyles*, 'new body consciousness', and a focus on fitness as the mark of success. Switzerland is a good example. The 1987 General Population Survey indicated a sharp reduction in the average amount of alcohol consumed daily by the entire Swiss population since 1981, with a special decline in the male population, the younger age groups, and the German-speaking cultural group. Fahrenkrug (1989) explains this trend by a growing proportion of the population switching to a more healthy lifestyle (stopping smoking, eating health food, exercising...) (see also Klingemann 1989). The change-of-normative-climate thesis also holds true for other health-related behaviour such as smoking (Abelin 1987).

The extent to which such changes in public opinion about health issues affects cohorts of substance users in the long run remains to be seen. Increased pressure and support by reference groups to change or to hide deviant behaviour, such as smoking, enjoying high cholesterol food, and preferring sleeping pills to herbal teas, can be plausibly assumed. At the same time, however, the missionary component of the new health ideology can produce individual reactance, lead to the formation or consolidation of subcultures, and consequently impede change.

One might add at this point that not only health-related values but also changes in *political thinking* can be related to patterns of substance behaviour. In longitudinal studies, period effects on illicit drug use during the 1960s and 1970s could be expected, based on the protest character of drug consumption in counter-cultures. Tightly knit sub-cultures offering a variety of arguments for the justification of drug use make it difficult for an individual to quit or, having quit, to maintain the individual strategies found to be effective in staying abstinent or in controlling consumption.

Comparing different cultures and countries, it becomes clear that the cultural setting determines the environmental conditions under which substance-related behaviour may change. Culture conflict of immigrants with the host society, constituting deviance, and the *acculturation* of ethnic groups are a classic theme since Sellin's work on culture-conflict and crime (1938). As a recent example, Kitano *et al.* (1992) compare the drinking practices and norms of Japanese in Japan and Japanese Americans. Drinking norms for the 16-year-olds and 60-year-olds are abstention-based and do not differ between the cultural settings. However, Japanese men hold more tolerant views of heavier drinking by men and are less tolerant of female drinking than Japanese men in America. The authors explain these findings by the rapid urbanization, industrialization, and the questioning of traditional values in Japan after World War II (*enculturation*) and the adoption by Japanese in America of more egalitarian norms towards female drinking (*acculturation*) Engs *et al.* (1990) discuss, in their recent study, the relative importance of *religion* and *culture* for social problems. Drawing upon the United States melting-pot assumption and the Canadian mosaic model they conclude: 'It appears that religious norms have greater influence in cohesive religious groups and culture has greater influence in less cohesive religious groups'. Cohesiveness in drinking norms largely transcends cultural differences in both countries; the Jewish and abstinence-oriented Protestant groups did not differ between countries.

Ethnic and religious influences on the drinking culture and consumption patterns in various countries are likely to increase in the future, given the rising numbers of migrants and a revival of regional thinking and ethnic consciousness. Identification with new groups and the adoption of value orientations play a large part in changing substance behaviour, as does a high degree of ethnic and cultural variety within society.

Mass media, average consumption, and motivation to change

Skog (1985) discusses the effects of the diffusion of norms and models on change in substance behaviour. This raises the issue of the effects of mass media communication on health behaviour and on the climate of consumption. Does the amount of advertising for alcoholic beverages, cigarettes, painkillers, and other substances affect total consumption? How do advertising or prevention messages affect the onset of addictive behaviour, motivation to change, and the maintenance of change?

Smart (1989) in his summary of the effects of bans on alcohol advertising comes to a negative answer to the first question. In his latest literature review on the subject Wilde (1991) points out that research in this area has been plagued by numerous methodological flaws and that mass communication prevention programmes for health and safety behaviour are rarely evaluated. Political bodies are often interested in only the immediate public-relation purpose of such campaigns and not in the assessment of long-term effects, which might yield disappointing results (Hauer 1990). The current discussions in the European Parliament as well as in Switzerland on banning advertising of tobacco and alcohol (Fahrenkrug 1992; Muster 1990) and the campaigns against illicit drugs exemplify how politically sensitive this topic is. More specific, however, are the effects on individuals and groups of *the interaction of media messages with psychological and social factors*: Burton *et al.* claim that, the lower the self-esteem of young people, the more susceptible they may be to tempting advertisements for cigarettes (Burton *et al.* 1989)—an interaction effect that favours first-time smoking.

Mass media can also strongly influence change in substance behaviour at later stages of a drug career or during the maintenance phase.

Supportive messages can reach substance users through significant others who improve their own coping skills at the same time ('the two-step flow of communication') and strengthen the users' motivation to quit. Self-help programmes, like the television-based smoking cessation pro-gramme reported by Danaher *et al.* (1984) in the Los Angeles area, are then perceived as helpful and serve to intensify attempts to quit. As the ESDA report has shown, many countries have stepped up their efforts during the last five years to launch mass media campaigns de-signed to reduce the marginalization of drug dependents in society, improve conditions for help-seeking, and help individuals maintain their resolution. However, the mass media still convey negative sterotypes, such as 'once an addict always an addict', which undermine motivation to change (Wong and Alexander, 1991). The finding of the Swiss study on natural recovery from heroin and alcohol addiction exemplifies this: most subjects, especially from the heroin group, tended to cover up their past and preferred not to tell their story of successful quitting; if they did, the reactions of others were still ambivalent (Klingemann 1992*a*).

Availability and perceived access—an issue not only for economists

Objective and perceived availability/access to licit and illicit drugs is determined by alcohol/drug policies, on taxation, outlet-density, drinking-age regulations, and the relative price of the substance, as well as changing personal income, which varies with the general economic situation (Österberg 1992). These conditions change the baseline for the substance user during the life course. *Heavy users* may substitute one expensive drug for a cheaper substance, illegally produce a substance, increase illegal income to maintain consumption habits, cut down on non drug-related items of other expenditure, or accept drug prescription/maintenance programmes. Similarly, as regards *young occasional users*, studies in Switzerland in 1986 and 1990 could detect no relationship between consumption trends and availability of illicit drugs; the effect of increased objective and subjective availability was counteracted by strong anti-drug norms and perceived health risks (Müller and Abbet 1991). Also in Switzerland, in the general population Leu and Lutz (1977) found that raising the prices of distilled spirits could lead to the substitution of fermented drinks for spirits, without reducing total con-sumption. Empirical estimates point to a totally price-inelastic demand for wine and a somewhat lower value for beer (Müller 1984).

An experiment in Switzerland aimed at young people with little money is the introduction of the so-called 'syrup-article' in several cantons, obliging pubs to offer at least one non-alcoholic beverage at a price lower than that of the cheapest alcoholic drink (Müller 1983). While politicians and the public welcome such measures to change the drinking environment of young people, other cantonal regulations, controlling outlet density (public-need clause—Bedürfnisklausel), are being gradually repealed.

DISCUSSION

Do environmental influences bring about changes in substance behaviour? The review of the empirical evidence presented here gives no simple answer. However, it seems to direct us to the following points:

1. Studies on relapse of **treated populations** show the salience of social factors and *commonalities* of risk situations *across the addictions*. The importance of the *interaction of interpersonal and intrapersonal* variables is emphasized. Social stability seems to be an important predictor of alcoholism outcome only in the short term, and indirect social pressure affects smokers most.

2. The latest studies on **natural recovery** from problem use of alcohol and heroin underline the importance of the *cognitive evaluation* of social and situational factors within a three-stage model. The prominent role of *social support*, particularly by the family, indicated by many studies, can be evaluated only with a more valid measurement of the support dimensions, and probably is specific to substance and stage.

3. **Longitudinal studies** provide little support for the assumption that *stressful life conditions* in themselves are associated with change. Status changes, such as the passage of juveniles to adulthood and from active professional life to retirement, influence, to some extent, the substance behaviour of individuals. A puzzling finding, however, is that the same social conditions under some circumstances seem to lead to an increase, and under others to a decrease, in substance use. The static single-event perspective seems to be less useful than a dynamic life-course perspective, which takes the functional meaning of events into consideration.

4. The growth of **treatment systems** does not necessarily promote change and may even jeopardize the individual's sense of self-efficacy. It is hypothesized that the trend in many countries towards low-threshold treatment, less coercion, the diversification of treatment efforts, forms of assisted spontaneous recovery, and

a more peaceful co-existence of the the social and medical model and self-help will promote change on a larger scale than before.

5. Finally, **social change** and institutions that affect the diffusion of substance-related norms and values in society make individual change more likely. *Healthy lifestyles* in the general population may encourage change, but at the extreme are likely to lead to reactance of the problem user. He refuses to be converted under great pressure and sees civil liberty in danger. The relationship between perceived access, objective availability, and individual change is more complex than usually assumed; there have been few group-specific studies on price and demand elasticity. Media messages influence the climate of consumption and determine the public stigma or positive image of various types of substance behaviour and consequently public views about how difficult or easy it is to change them.

This tentative summary needs to be kept in perspective. Differences in design and methods of studies, and frequently missing detailed background information (particularly if studies are presented in journal articles), make a meta-analysis very difficult. Context and system conditions, such as cultural factors, must be included, but complicate the picture. All this is rather a standard conclusion of most reviews of this type and comes as no surprise. However, the point about the significance of context effects is not just another variable within a causal model of change; rather, it leads to a more comprehensive view of the scientific exploration of change in substance behaviour.

We have shown above that the development of treatment ideologies and concepts, such as the disease paradigm, reflected to some extent broader changes in social values. Going one step further, it will be necessary to consider societal influence on the scientific communities undertaking addiction research (for example Weingart 1983). Funding policies, ethical requirements, and political ideologies obviously guide and channel research efforts to a large extent. Hence, changing modes of research financing may determine the extent to which specific types of substance behaviour are investigated, the possibilities of *interdisciplinary* research, and the conditions for both medical researchers and social and behavioural researchers in the addiction field. Problems of ethnocentric views and lack of communication within scientific communities are another bias that must be allowed for in assessing empirical evidence about the explanatory power of physiological, intrapersonal, and environmental factors. An excellent example is the review of psychosocial correlates of adolescent substance use by Moncher *et al.* (1991).

Among the 80 studies included in the review there are only seven from outside the United States and one from a non-anglophone country, excluding completely, for example, the WHO cross-national surveys on health behaviour in school-age children, conducted already for the second time in 15 countries. The analysis of citation networks in the field would probably yield interesting supplementary results. Of course, whether treatment providers and policy makers use these results to promote individual change or merely to defend their *professional interests and resist change in their professional behaviour, is another question. The cutting of state funds for studies of natural recovery in the German Land Hessen is an interesting case in point (Happel 1986).

REFERENCES

Abelin, T. (1987). *Immer weniger Raucher*. Pressekonferenz, Bern.

Baar, M. and O'Connor, S. (1985). Relapse in alcoholism: New perspectives. *American Journal of Orthopsychiatry*, **55**, 570–6.

Barrera, M. Jr (1986). Distinctions between social support concepts, measures, and models. *American Journal of Community Psychology*, **14**, 413.

Blackwell, J. S. (1983). Drifting, controlling and overcoming: Opiate users who avoid becoming chronically dependent. *Journal of Drug Issues*, **13**, 219–35.

Blaszczynski, A., McConaghy, N., and Frankova, A. (1991). Control versus abstinence in the treatment of pathological gambling: A two to nine year follow-up. *British Journal of Addiction*, **86**, 299–306.

Brady, M. (1993). Giving away the grog: ethnography of aboriginal drinkers who quit without help. *Drug and Alcohol Review*, **12**, 401–11.

Brennan, P. L., and Moos, R. H. (1991). Functioning life context and help-seeking among late-onset problem drinkers: comparisons with nonproblem and early-onset problem drinkers. *British Journal of Addiction*, **86**, 1139–50.

Brown, J. D. (1991). The professional ex-: Or exiting the deviant career. *The Sociological Quarterly*, **32**, 219–30.

Brownell, K. D., Marlatt G. A., Lichtenstein, E., and Wilson G. T. (1986). Understanding and preventing relapse. *American Psychologist*, **41**, 765–82.

Burton, D., Sussman, S., Hansen, W. B., and Johnson C. (1989). Image attributions and smoking intentions among seventh grade students. *Journal of Applied Social Psychology*, **19**, 658–64.

Clarke, M., Farid, B., and Romaniuk, H. (1990). Occupational risk factors in alcoholism. *British Journal of Addiction*, **85**, 1611–14.

Danaher, B. G., Berkanovic, E., and Gerber, B. (1984). Mass media based health behavior change: Televised smoking cessation program. *Addictive Behaviors*, **9**, 245–53.

Dohrenwend, B. P., Link, B. G., Kern R., Shrout, P. E., and Markowitz, J. (1987). Measuring life events: the problem of variability within event categories. In *Psychiatric epidemiology: progress and prospects*, (ed. B. Cooper), pp. 103–19. Croom Helm, London.

Emrick, C. D. A. (1975). A review of psychologically oriented treatment of alcoholism: II. The relative effectiveness of different treatment approaches and the effectiveness of treatment versus no treatment. *Journal of Studies on Alcohol*, **36**, 88–108.

Engs, R. C., Hanson, D. J., Gliksman, L,. and Smythe, C. (1990). Influence of religion and culture on drinking behaviours: A test of hypotheses between Canada and the USA. *British Journal of Addiction*, **85**, 1475–82

Fahrenkrug, H. (1989). Swiss drinking habits: results of surveys in 1975, 1981 and 1987. *Contemporary Drug Problems*, **16**, 201–25.

Fahrenkrug, H. (1992). Legislations actuelles sur la publicité concernant le vin et les spiritueux en Europe Centrale (Suisse, Allemagne, Benelux). (Paper presented at *Il Centenario de la Estación Enológica de Haro (La Rioja)*, 11–13 February. Bilbao.

Foote A. and Erfurt, J. C. (1991). Effects of EAP follow-up on prevention of relapse among substance abuse clients. *Journal of Studies on Alcohol*, **52**, 241–8.

Goor van de, L. A. M., Knibbe, R. A., and Drop, M. J. (1990). Adolescent drinking behavior: An observational study of the influence of situational factors on adolescent drinking rates. *Journal of Studies on Alcohol*, **51**, 548–55.

Gorman, D. M. and Peters, T. J. (1990). Types of life events and the onset of alcohol dependence. *British Journal of Addiction*, **85**, 71–9.

Graeven, D. B. and Graeven, K. A. (1983). Treated and untreated addicts: Factors associated with participation in treatment and cessation of heroin use. *Journal of Drug Issues*, **13**, 207–18.

Green G., Macintyre, S., West, P., and Ecob, R. (1991). Like parent like child? Associations between drinking and smoking behaviour of parents and their children. *British Journal of Addiction*, **86**, 745–58.

Hagan, J. (1991). Destiny and drift: Subcultural preferences status attainments, and the risks and rewards of youth. *American Sociological Review*, **56**, 567–82.

Happel, H.-V. (1986). Ausstieg aus der Drogenabhängigkeit am Beispiel der Selbstheiler. Projektbeschreibung. *Suchtgefahren*, **32**, 367–8.

Hauer E. (1990). The behaviour of public bodies and the delivery of road safety. *Proceedings, Enforcement and Rewarding, International Road Safety Symposium*, pp. 134–8. Sept. 19–21. Copenhagen.

Heather, N. (1986). Change without therapists: The use of self-help manuals by problem drinkers. In *Treating addictive behaviors*. (ed. W. R. Miller and Nick Heather), pp. 331–59. Plenum Publishing Corporation, New York.

Jung, J. (1986). How significant others cope with problem drinkers. *The International Journal of the Addictions*, **21**, 813–17.

Kail, B. L. and Litwak, E. (1989). Family friends and neighbors: the role of primary groups in preventing the misuse of drugs. *The Journal of Drug Issues*, **19**, 261–81.

Kendell, R. E. and Staton, M. (1966). The fate of untreated alcoholics. *Quarterly Journal of Studies on Alcohol*, **27**, 30.

Kitano, H. H. L., Chi, I., Rhee, S., and Lubben, J. E. (1992). Norms and alcohol consumption: Japanese in Japan, Hawaii and California. *Journal of Studies on Alcohol*, **53**, 33–9.

Klein H. and Pittman, D. J. (1990). Social occasions and the perceived appropriateness of consuming different alcoholic beverages. *Journal of Studies on Alcohol*, **51**, 59–67.

Klingemann, H. K.-H. (1984). Voluntarism and professional intervention in alcohol problems as interdependent problem-solving potentials: The case of Switzerland. Paper presented at the IGCAS meeting *Societal Responses to Alcohol Problems and Development of Treatment Systems*. Lindgoe, Sweden.

Klingemann, H. K.-H. (1988). Der soziale Kontext von Autoremissionen bei problematischem Alkoholkonsum. *Medizin Mensch Gesellschaft*, **13**, 123–31.

Klingemann, H. K.-H. (1989). Supply and demand-oriented measures of alcohol policy in Switzerland—current trends and drawbacks. *Health Promotion*, **4**, 305–15.

Klingemann, H. K.-H. (1990). Initiierung und Verlauf von Autoremissionsprozessen bei Abhängigkeitsproblemen. *Schweizerische Fachstelle für Alkoholprobleme*. Lausanne.

Klingemann, H. K.-H. (1991). The motivation for change from problem alcohol and heroin use. *British Journal of Addiction*, **86**, 727–44

Klingemann, H. K.-H. (1992a). Coping and maintenance strategies of spontaneous remitters from problem use of alcohol and heroin in Switzerland. *International Journal of Addictions*, **27**, 1359–88.

Klingemann, H. K.-H. (1992b). *European Summary on Drug Abuse: Report*. World Health Organization, Copenhagen.

Klingemann, H. K.-H. (1992c). Everyday definitions of deviant behavior. Computer-assisted content analysis of lay concepts of alcohol and drug problems, delinquency and youth problems. In *Textanalyse. Anwendungen der computerunterstützten Inhaltsanalyse* (ed. C. Züll, M. Mohler, and A. Geis), pp. 105–29. Westdeutscher Verlag. Opladen.

Klingemann, H. K.-H. and Takala, J.-P. (1987). International studies of the development of alcohol treatment systems—a research agenda for the future. *Contemporary Drug Problems*, **14**, 1–13.

Klingemann, H. K.-H. et al. (1992). The role of alcohol treatment in a consensus democracy—the case of the Swiss Confederation. In *Cure, care, or control: Alcoholism treatment in sixteen countries* (ed. H. Klingemann, J.-P. Takala, and G. Hunt), pp. 151–72. State University of New York Press, Albany.

Lando, H. A., Pirie, P. L., McGovern, P. G., Pechacek, T. F., Swim, J., and Loken B. (1991). A comparison of self-help approaches to smoking cessation. *Addictive Behaviors*, **16**, 183–93.

Leu, R. and Lulz (1977). *Oekonomische Aspekte des Alkoholismus in der Schweiz*. Schulthess, Zurich.

Mäkelä K. (1991). Social and cultural preconditions of Alcoholics Anonymous

(AA) and factors associated with the strength of AA. *British Journal of Addiction*, **86**, 1405–13.

Marlatt, G. A. and Gordon, J. R. (1980). Determinants of relapse: Implications for the maintenance of behavior change. In *Behavioral medicine: Changing health lifestyles* (ed. P. O. Davidson and S. M. Davidson), pp. 411–52. Brunner/Mazel, New York.

Marlatt, G. A. and Gordon J. R. (1985). *Relapse prevention: Maintenance strategies in addictive behavior change*. Guilford, New York.

Mayer, K. U. and Huinink, J. (1990). Alters-, Perioden- und Kohorteneffekte in der Analyse von Lebensverläufen oder: Lexis ade? *Kölner Zeitschrift für Soziologie und Sozialpsychologie*, **31**, 442–59.

Miller, W. R. (1986). Haunted by the Zeitgeist: Reflections on contrasting treatment goals and concepts of alcoholism in Europe and the United States. In *Alcohol and culture* (ed. T. Babor). Academy of Sciences, New York.

Miller W. R. and Hester, R. K. (1986). The effectiveness of alcoholism treatment: What research reveals. In *Treating addictive behaviors: processes of change* (ed. W. R. Miller, and N. K. Heather), pp. 121–73. Plenum, New York.

Moncher, M. S., Holden, G. W., and Schinke, S. P. (1991). Psychosocial correlates of adolescent substance use: A review of current etiological constructs. *The International Journal of the Addictions*, **26**, 377–414.

Moos, R. H. and Sindle, R. W. Jr (1990). Stressful life circumstances: concepts and measures. In *Stress medicine*, Vol. 6, pp. 171–8. John Wiley & Sons, Chichester.

Müller, R. (1983). Le débat d'actualité: le prix de la bière dans la constellation des causes de 'l'alcoolisme des jeunes'. *Drogalkohol*, **2**, 49–51.

Müller, R. (1984). Die Lenkung des Angebotes alkoholischer Getränke als primärpräventive Massnahme gegenüber Alkoholproblemen. *Schweizerische Fachstelle für Alkoholprobleme*. Lausanne.

Müller R. and Abbet, J.-P. (1991). Veränderungen im Konsum legaler und illegaler Drogen bei Jugendlichen. *Schweizerische Fachstelle für Alkoholprobleme*, Lausanne.

Muster, E. (1990). Publicity for alcoholic beverages—the risks of European harmonization. Paper presented at the *35th International Institute ICAA, Section Alcohol Policy*, Berlin.

Needle, R., McCubbin, H., Wilson, M., Reineck, R., Lazar, A., and Mederer, H. (1986). Interpersonal influences in adolescent drug use—the role of older siblings, parents, and peers. *The International Journal of the Addictions*, **21**, 739–66.

Noschis, K. (1988/89). Testing a self-help instrument with early-risk alcohol consumers in general practice: A progress report. *Contemporary Drug Problems*, **15**, 365–81.

Oei, T. P. S. and Hallam, J. (1991). Behavioral strategies used by long-term successful self-quitters. *The International Journal of the Addictions*, **26**, 993–1002.

Öjesjö L. (1991). Alcohol addiction and biography. Paper presented at *17th*

Annual Epidemiology Symposium, Kettil Bruun Society for Social and Epidemiological Research on Alcohol, June 9–14, Sigtuna.

Orcutt, J. D. (1987). Differential association and marijuana use: A closer look at Sutherland (with a little help from Becker). *Criminology*, **25**, 341–58.

Österberg E. (1992). Effects of alcohol control measures on alcohol consumption. *The International Journal of the Addictions*, **27**, 209–25.

Pagel, M. D., Erdly, W. W., and Becker, J. (1987). Social networks: we get by with (and in spite of) a little help from our friends. *Journal of Personality and Social Psychology*, **53**, 793–804.

Peele, S. (1989). *Diseasing of America: Addiction treatment out of control*. Lexington Books, Lexington, Massachusetts.

Peele, S. (1990–91). What works in addiction treatment and what doesn't: Is the best therapy no therapy? *The International Journal of the Addictions*, **25**, 1409–19.

Power C. and Estaugh, V. (1990*a*). The role of family formation and dissolution in shaping drinking behaviour in early adulthood. *British Journal of Addiction*, **85**, 521–30.

Power C. and Estaugh, V. (1990*b*). Employment and drinking in early adulthood: A longitudinal perspective. *British Journal of Addiction*, **85**, 487–94.

Romelsjö A., Lazarus, N. B., Kaplan, G. A., and Cohen, R. D. (1991). The relationship between stressful life situations and changes in alcohol consumption in a general population sample. *British Journal of Addiction*, **86**, 157–69.

Sandahl, C. (1984). Determinants of relapse among alcoholics: A cross-cultural replication study. *The International Journal of the Addictions*, **19**, 833–48.

Saunders, W. M. and Kershaw, M. D. (1979). Spontaneous remission from alcoholism—a community study. *British Journal of Addiction*, **74**, 251–65.

Sellin, Th. (1938). Culture conflict and crime. *Social Science Research Council Bulletin*, **41**, 63–70.

Sjöberg, L. (1983). Value change and relapse following a decision to quit or reduce smoking. *Scandinavian Journal of Psychology*, **24**, 37–48.

Skog, O.-J. (1985). The collectivity of drinking cultures: A theory of the distribution of alcohol consumption. *British Journal of Addiction*, **80**, 83–99.

Smart, R. G. (1975/76). Spontaneous recovery in alcoholics: A review and analysis of the available research. *Drug and Alcohol Dependence*, **1**, 277–85.

Smart, R. G. (1989). Is the postwar drinking binge ending? Cross-national trends in per capital alcohol consumption. *British Journal of Addiction*, **84**, 743–8.

Sobell, L. C., Cunningham, J. A., Sobell, M. B., and Toneatto, T. (1991). A life span perspective on natural recovery (self-change) from alcohol problems. In *Addictive behaviors across the lifespan: prevention, treatment, and policy issues* (ed. J. S. Baer, G. A. Marlatt, and R. J. McMahon), pp. 34–66. Sage Publications, Beverly Hills, CA.

Sobell, L. C., Sobell, M. B., and Toneatto, T. (1992). Recovery from alcohol problems without treatment. In *Self-control and addictive behaviors* (ed. N. Heather, W. R. Miller, and J. Greeley), pp. 198–242. Maxwell Macmillan, New York.

Sobell, L. C., Sobell, M. B., Toneatto, T., and Leo, G. I. (1993). What triggers the resolution of alcohol problems without treatment? *Alcoholism: Clinical and Experimental Research*, **17**, 217–24.

Spinatsch, M. and Chilvers, C. (1991). Die Lebensverhältnisse von Alkoholabhängigen nach stationärer Behandlung. *Schweizerische Fachstelle für Alkoholprobleme*. Lausanne.

Stall, R. (1983). An examination of spontaneous remission from problem drinking in the bluegrass region of Kentucky. *Journal of Drug Issues*, **13**, 191–206.

Stall, R. (1986*a*). Change and stability in quantity and frequency of alcohol use among aging males: A 19-year follow-up study. *British Journal of Addiction*, **81**, 537–44.

Stall, R. (1986*b*). Respondent-identified reasons for change and stability in alcohol consumption as a concomitant of the aging process. In *Anthropology and Epidemiology* (ed. C. R. Janes *et al.*), pp. 275–301. D. Reidel Publishing Company, Lancaster.

Stall, R. and Biernacki, P. (1986). Spontaneous remission from the problematic use of substances: An inductive model derived from a comparative analysis of the alcohol opiate, tobacco, and food/obesity literatures. *The International Journal of the Addictions*, **21**, 1–23.

Tecklenburg, U. (1986). The present-day alcohol treatment system in Switzerland: a historical perspective. *Contemporary Drug Problems*, **13**, 555–83.

Temple, M. T., Middleton Fillmore, K, Hartka, E. Johnston, B., Leino, E. V., and Motoyoshi, M. (1991). The collaborative alcohol-related longitudinal project. *British Journal of Addiction*, **86**, 1269–81.

Trice, H. M. and Sonnenstuhl, W. J. (1990). On the construction of drinking norms in work organizations. *Journal of Studies on Alcohol*, **51**, 201–20.

Tuchfeld, B. S. (1981). Spontaneous remission in alcoholics. *Journal of Studies on Alcohol*, **42**, 626–41.

Tucker, J. A. and Gladsjo, J. A. (1993). Help-seeking and recovery by problem drinkers: characteristics of drinkers who attend A. A. formal treatment, or achieve problem resolution alone. *Addictive Behaviours*, **18**, 529–42.

Vaillant, G. E. (1983). *The natural history of alcoholism: Causes, patterns, and paths to recovery*. Harvard University Press, Cambridge, Massachusetts.

Waldorf, D. (1983). The social-psychological processes of control and recovery from substance abuse. *Journal of Drug Issues*, **13**, 189–90.

Waldorf, D. and Biernacki, P. (1979). Natural recovery from heroin addiction: a review of the incidence literature. *Journal of Drug Issues*, **9**, 281–9.

Waldorf, D. and Biernacki, P. (1981). The natural recovery from opiate addiction: some preliminary findings. *Journal of Drug Issues*, **11**, 61–74.

Weingart, P. (1983). Verwissenschaftlichung der Gesellschaft—Politisierung der Wissenschaft. *Zeitschrift für Soziologie*, **3**, 225–41.

Wheaton, B. (1990). Life transitions, role histories, and mental health. *American Sociological Reviews*, **55**, 209–23.

Wilde, G. J. S. (1991). Effects of mass media communications upon health and safety habits of individuals: an overview of issues and evidence. *Addiction*, **88**, 983–96.

Wong, L. S. and Alexander, B. K. (1991). 'Cocaine-related' deaths: Media coverage in the war on drugs. *Journal of Drug Issues*, **21**, 105–19.

Zimmerman, R. S. and Connor, C. (1989). Health promotion in context: The effects of significant others on health behavior change. *Health Education Quarterly*, **16**, 57–75.

9

Economic influences on change in population and personal substance behaviour

CHRISTINE GODFREY

INTRODUCTION

Changes in the consumption of alcohol and tobacco have considerable economic importance. For example, in the United Kingdom alcohol consumption accounted for 6.3 per cent and tobacco consumption 2.6 per cent of total consumers' expenditure in 1990. The markets for illegal drugs in the United Kingdom are estimated to be much smaller. For example, in 1984 the expenditure on heroin was estimated at only 3–6 per cent of the level of tobacco consumption (Wagstaff and Maynard 1988). For other countries, whether major suppliers or consumers, the illegal drug economy is much larger. Understanding economic influences on the consumption levels of all substances can provide useful insights for predicting changes in substance use and the need for service responses.

For both legal and illegal goods, market transactions between the consumers and suppliers determine consumption, and substance use can be affected by changing the factors influencing both groups. Many resources have been devoted to restricting the supply of illegal drugs. This has involved attempting to increase the costs facing the producers and dealers, by enforcement activities in supplying and consuming countries, and attempting to increase the rewards from other activities, by crop substitution activities. In contrast, more attention has been focused on altering consumption, through prevention policies directed at individual consumers, for legal drugs.

In this chapter, economic models of factors influencing both population and individual substance behaviour and some of the empirical results from applying these models are reviewed. Lack of data has restricted economic analysis of illegal drug markets, hence alcohol and tobacco studies will form the main focus of the chapter.

In most countries, alcohol and tobacco are subject to special taxes and both governments and economists have been interested in estimating changes in total consumption and consequent changes in tax revenue. The empirical work undertaken at a population level is considered in the following section. Different models and different influences can be explored with data on individuals and this work is described in the third section of the chapter. Much of the modelling of substance use undertaken by economists has involved similar analyses to that applied to most other goods. There has, however, been a body of research which has attempted to devise specific models to account for addictive behaviour and to examine the implications of this behaviour on the measured importance of economic factors as determinants of changes in substance use. This work is considered in the fourth section. The role of suppliers' influences on substance use and the policy process are briefly discussed in the fifth section. Finally, some conclusions are drawn on the role of economic factors in the process of changing patterns of substance use, the policy implications of existing work, and the areas where economic analysis could be usefully extended in both legal and illegal markets.

ECONOMIC FACTORS AND CHANGES IN POPULATION LEVELS OF SUBSTANCE USE

Consumers have to make choices about the goods they wish to purchase. Prices of the substances, the prices of other goods, and available income are the economic factors likely to affect consumption decisions. Data on these variables tend to be readily available at the national or state level for alcohol and tobacco, although even official estimates may underestimate consumption because of smuggling and home production. Some idea of the influence of economic factors can be gained from examining trends over time of these variables. For example, in the United Kingdom the trends in the consumption of cigarettes per head and trends in cigarette prices relative to other goods seem to move inversely with one another, as shown in Fig. 9.1. Hence in periods when prices rise, consumption tends to fall. For alcohol this inverse pattern can only be observed if the price series is adjusted to show changes relative to income (Fig. 9.2). Falls in relative prices during the 1960s and 1970s accompanied by growth in incomes are two of the causes for the sharp increase in alcohol consumption during this period.

While an examination of trends gives a useful indication of possible relationships, more rigorous analysis is required to examine the

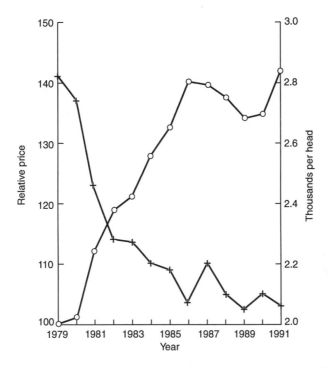

FIG. 9.1 Cigarette consumption and relative prices. +, number (thousands) per head for the population aged 15 and over. o Refer to the relative price— relative to the 'All Items' index (1979 = 100); Figures for 1991 for 3 quarters only). (Source: Central Statistical Office.)

importance of these factors. Economists rarely have access to experimental data and so, in general, have to build and estimate models which take into account all the relevant factors. The data used for the population studies can be the time-series type used in the figures. Other studies have compared data across countries, and in some countries, mainly the United States, differences in legislation, taxes, and prices across different parts of the country have allowed models to be estimated using pooled time-series and state, cross-sectional data. Different data allow different influences to be examined. Social changes and influences are unlikely to be detected using simple time series, but may differ within countries. In some of the cross-national studies the effects of different legislative approaches to alcohol and tobacco control have been of interest.

The main influences considered in population studies in addition to price and income are advertising, regulations, especially availability, and,

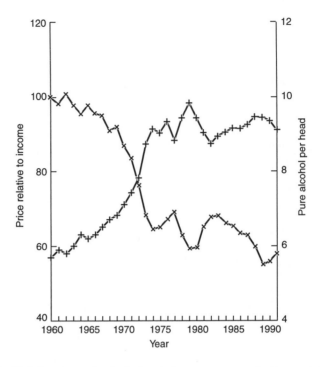

FIG. 9.2 Retail price of alcohol relative to personal disposable income (crosses), and consumption of pure alcohol per head of population aged 15 or over +,−1960 to 1991. (Source: Customs and Excise; Centre for Health Economics database.)

for tobacco, health information. Reviews of these studies indicate a divergence of findings with the data, the specification of the models, and estimation methods used (see, for example, Godfrey 1989; Lewit 1989; Osterberg, 1991; Ponicki, 1990). It may be expected that influences would vary between countries. It is not possible to give details of all studies, but some of the findings concerning major influences and the implications of the empirical results are considered below.

Price

Economic models of alcohol and tobacco demand are generally estimated using multiple regression techniques. The functional forms of relationships, that is whether the equations are estimated as linear, logarithmic, or other mathematical forms, vary as does the inclusion or exclusion of certain variables. Model differences make it difficult to simply compare results, but economists compute elasticities from regression estimates of parameters. The elasticity is an index which measures the sensitivity of demand and because it is unit free can be computed and compared for various models. A price elasticity can be defined in the following way. If price changes by a small amount, with all the other variables in the demand function being held constant, then demand will also change. The price elasticity is defined as the ratio of the proportionate change in demand to the proportionate change in price. Roughly speaking, an own-price elasticity for tobacco of −0.5 would imply that a 1 per cent increase in the price of tobacco, with all other factors being fixed, would lead to a 0.5 per cent drop in the demand for tobacco. Price elasticity estimates are generally negative because if prices rise consumers will tend to buy less of the good. In contrast, income elasticities are generally positive because if incomes rise consumers can afford to buy more of the good.

In the doubly logarithmic functional form, where both the dependent variable, alcohol or tobacco consumption, and the independent variables, such as price and income, are expressed as logarithms, the elasticities are constant over the whole range of observations. This may not always be a realistic assumption. For example, it may be expected that as the number of smokers falls then so may the price elasticity estimate, as those remaining smokers are less responsive to price changes.

Price elasticities may also be expected to vary with the type of goods. The demand for luxury (and new) goods would be expected to be more responsive to price changes than necessities. Inelastic price elasticities are those between 0 and −1.0.

For the UK and the USA, the majority of studies have indicated that tobacco consumption is price inelastic. Estimates for the UK vary between −1.05 to 0, but −0.5 was thought to be a reasonable midpoint estimate and was the official Treasury figure for a number of years (Godfrey 1989). A comparison of a number of models using a common data set from 1956 to 1984 yielded a price elasticity estimate of −0.56 for the consumption measure of the weight of tobacco in cigarettes (Godfrey and Maynard, 1988). More recently the official estimate has been revised downwards to −0.3.

American results based on time series or pooled time-series and cross-sections of states give estimates of tobacco price elasticities between −0.14 and −1.23 with −0.7 being used by the Tobacco Institute to calculate tax effects (Lewit 1989). Similar price effects have been found elsewhere amongst developed countries, but there have been few studies of developing countries where cigarette consumption has been rising rapidly.

Examining the effects of price on alcohol consumption is more complicated because of the need to consider beverages separately rather than attempting to estimate a single model of alcohol consumption (Walsh 1982). It would be expected that price elasticities of different beverages would be linked to consumption levels, with the most popular beverages being the least responsive to changes in price. This hypothesis does seem to be supported by empirical evidence. In the UK, for example, price elasticity estimates for beer, the most popular beverage, have generally been below −0.5. Drinking preferences do change, however, and the share of beer consumption has been falling. In 1965 beer consumption, in terms of pure litres of alcohol was 72.7 per cent of total consumption, but this share had fallen to 55.3 per cent in 1990. Beer prices also rose sharply, and compared to 1979 had risen to be 40 per cent higher than the general inflation rate by 1991. These sharp price increases and possible changes in taste may have been expected to result in different price estimates. Both a new Treasury estimate and results from a study using data up to 1989 (Glenn and Carr-Hill 1991) give higher estimates of beer price elasticity than previously at −1.0 and −0.8, respectively. Glen and Carr-Hill also suggest that beer and lager consumption should be considered separately.

Early studies of spirits and wine demand in the UK gave higher price elasticities than for beer, but they were highly variable and it was difficult to find summary figures. There has been a recent change in UK drinking habits, with an increase in wine drinking. The studies using the most recent data seem to indicate that price elasticities for all beverages are closer to each other. For example, the Treasury estimate for wine is −1.1 and for spirits is −0.9.

In the United States and Canada a similar pattern of lower beer price elasticities to other beverages emerges, although Ponicki (1990) gives a higher best guess estimate for beer at −0.6 compared to −0.2 for Canada. His best guess estimates for spirits are −1.0 and −0.7 and for wine −1.3 and −0.6, for the USA and Canada, respectively.

Most other countries will have access to price elasticity estimates either from official sources or from research studies, but only a few are published more widely. Also some studies use alternative time-series techniques to investigate price effects. For example, Ahtola *el al.* (1986) used Baysian methods to consider trends in price (and income) elasticities in Finland from 1955 to 1980. They found that there were clear downward trends in both price and income elasticities (calculated on total alcohol figures) at a time when the country was becoming more affluent.

It is clearly more difficult to obtain time-series data on both consumption and prices of illegal drugs in order to calculate price elasticities. Available estimates have to use indirect methods to estimate consumption levels (Wagstaff 1989). Despite an often widespread view that drug users would not respond to changes in prices, available analysis from US data suggests that the price elasticity for heroin in the 1970s was approximately -0.25 (Silverman and Spruill 1977). Using survey estimates and questions about how much students would be willing to pay for drugs, Nisbet and Vakil (1972) found price elasticity estimates for marihuana in the range -0.40 to -1.51.

Cross-price effects

It is not only the price of the goods in question relative to all other goods which is likely to affect demand, but also the prices of any substitutes or complements. It is obviously important to know if increasing the price of one substance acts to decrease all substance use or results in consumers switching from one substance to another. In simple economic models, which estimate the demand for each good separately, few significant cross-price effects have been found for alcohol or tobacco (Godfrey 1986*a*). Another method of estimating demand equations is to estimate a system or sub-system of demand equations, taking into account the interrelationships between goods.

A number of studies have used this approach to estimate subsystems of demand for different alcohol beverages (Clements and Johnson 1983; Duffy 1987; Salvananthan 1988). It may be expected that alcoholic drinks would be substitutes for each other and that if, for example, the price of beer increased the demand for wines and spirits would rise. This would imply positive cross-price effects. Most empirical estimates suggest that cross-price effects are small and insignificant. As with own-price figures, these estimates have to be treated with some caution and may change with prosperity or drinking habits. Across many developed countries there has been some evidence of a harmonization of drinking patterns, with countries adding new habits to established ones. For example, countries which traditionally have been mainly episodic beer drinkers have adopted the habit of drinking wine with meals (Sparrow *et al.* 1989). If drinking habits are associated with different social circumstances then it may be expected that estimates of cross-price effects will continue to be small. Further studies using the most recent data will be needed to test this hypothesis.

Few economic studies have considered the interactions between different substances. An exception is a study by Jones (1989*a*) where a subsystem of demand equations for tobacco, beer, wines, and spirits was estimated using UK data for the period 1964–1983. Tobacco was found to be a complement to all four types of alcoholic drink with the results suggesting, for example, that a 1 per cent increase in tobacco prices would lead to a decrease in beer and wine consumption of 0.2

per cent and a decrease of spirits and cider consumption of 0.5 per cent, other factors remaining unchanged. Individual survey data do indicate that smoking and heavy drinking behaviour are linked and could account for a large proportion of expenditure of some individuals (Godfrey and Posnett 1988) which may help explain these results.

For illicit drugs the possibility of substitution has been more widely debated, and although estimates are not available several authors have suggested that own price elasticities may vary with prices, legal enforcement activities, and the availability of other substances (see the review in Wagstaff and Maynard 1988). Wagstaff and Maynard suggest a demand curve where demand is responsive to price at low and very high prices but is completely inelastic at medium prices. It is hypothesized that at lower prices 'non-addicts' curtail consumption, while at very high prices 'addicts' find it difficult to finance habits from criminal activities and reduce consumption, seek treatment, or switch to lower priced drugs. The evidence of such responses would be difficult to obtain. Also, it is clear that street prices for different substances show considerable variation and often cheaper alternatives exist for currently 'fashionable' substances. It is clear that consumers' behaviour in the illicit markets is as complex as for drinking, and there are considerable dangers in applying simplistic economic models especially to guide enforcement activities.

Changing prices and taxation

Taxation issues have meant that estimates of price effects for alcohol and tobacco goods have received a great deal of attention from both economists and health policy analysts. While a review of price effects, as above, reveals that not all estimates are large, it is known that increasing prices will be effective in reducing population levels of consumption. The evidence on effectiveness for other policies, such as prevention or treatment, is not always available. Tax systems differ but in most countries part of the tax is set in monetary terms. This means that unless taxes are uprated they lose value with inflation and this can result in a downward pressure on price. Understanding how taxes are set and how they can be changed has, therefore, received a lot of attention from policy analysts who are concerned with population levels of substance use.

Taxes are not the only determinant of prices and supply factors may influence prices. For example, the price of beer in the UK has been increasing much faster than inflation, even in years, such as 1989, when the level of excise duty was not changed in the annual Budget. Also, manufacturers or retailers may choose to curtail prevention policies by absorbing some tax increases and not raising prices. The ability of manufacturers and retailers to influence price changes depends on the proportion of tax in price. The higher this proportion, the smaller is the suppliers ability to influence prices. In the UK the total tax as a proportion of price was, in 1991: 76 per cent for a packet of cigarettes; 68 per cent for a bottle of whisky; 57 per cent for a bottle of table wine; and 33 per cent for a pint of beer. In general, countries attempt to favour home-produced goods in their alcohol and tobacco taxation policies and discriminate against imported goods (Powell 1989).

Another factor influencing the use of taxes as a public health measure is the historic pattern of taxes. A policy of relating alcohol taxes to their alcohol content may seem sensible in health terms. However, the rate of duty per litre of pure alcohol is much heavier for spirits (£18.96 in 1991) than for beer (£10.08). Changes in tax policy face considerable impediments including political factors, macro-economic policy concerns, supplier groups lobbying, and, within Europe, the Single Market policy (Godfrey and Harrison 1990).

Income

While tax policy may give some control over prices, income changes are outside public health policy influence. As greater income allows individuals to buy more of all goods, it would be expected that as general prosperity rises population levels of substance use would also increase. Income elasticity estimates are available from the same studies as were reviewed for the price effects. Tobacco income elasticities have been generally found to be positive and below 1, ranging in the UK, for example, between 0.12 and 0.68 (Godfrey 1989). The current Treasury income elasticity estimate is 0.3, which would suggest that a rise of 1 per cent of disposable income would increase tobacco consumption by 0.3 per cent, other things being equal.

Estimates of alcohol income elasticities have generally been much higher than those for tobacco, especially for beverages considered as luxuries in the country concerned. In the UK, for example, income elasticities estimated from single equation studies have varied between 0.60 and 2.76 for spirits and 0.49 to 2.53 for wine (Godfrey 1989). Results from system estimates of demand, which refer to total expenditure rather than income, have generally yielded estimates in the same ranges (Jones 1989a). Income elasticities for beer in the UK have been found to be lower than for other beverages, falling between 0.12 and 1.1.

For the USA and Canada, Ponicki's best guess elasticity estimates are smaller for beer (0.4 and 0.1 respectively) than for spirits (0.6 and 0.4) and wine (1.3 and 0.3). These figures seem considerably lower than those for the UK. Recent official estimates in the UK have also been revised downwards with new estimates of income elasticity of 0.9 for spirits and 1.6 for wine compared to previous estimates of 1.8 and 2.6. Weighting the new estimates by expenditure share would suggest that overall alcohol consumption in the UK would increase 1.1 per cent for every 1 per cent increase in disposable income, other factors remaining unchanged. For the UK, at least, increasing prosperity is likely to lead to more alcohol problems.

Advertising

The debate about econometric evidence on the effect of advertising on alcohol and tobacco consumption has been particularly fierce. Many demand studies have included a term measuring alcohol expenditure or the volume of alcohol messages. Both health and industry lobbies have used different studies to support arguments for more or less advertising restrictions. In assessing this area it is necessary to first critically review the available studies and then consider their implications for guiding policy decisions about advertising restrictions.

Commentaries about divergent results between studies have concentrated on the significance of advertising terms. Statistical significance can only be judged, however, if a model is well specified, and many of the early studies of tobacco were not subjected to the battery of tests which have recently become accepted as good econometric practice (Godfrey 1986b). Also, it is important to note that an insignificant variable does not necessarily mean that a variable has no influence but only that its effects cannot be precisely estimated.

The available empirical evidence on the effects of variations of the level of advertising on alcohol and tobacco consumption is mixed, but most of the available elasticity estimates are small in magnitude, usually less than 0.1 (Smart 1988; Chetwynd *et al.* 1988; Godfrey and Maynard 1988; Godfrey 1989). These types of estimates would suggest that a 1 per cent decrease in advertising would result in less than 0.1 per cent decrease in consumption.

There are problems with these type of estimates, however, especially when attempting to forecast the effects of changing advertising regulations. Generally available advertising figures do not include all forms of advertising and marketing. In the UK only data on TV and press advertising are available to independent researchers. Nor can these econometric models be reliably used to forecast major shifts in policy such as an advertising ban. The calculated effects of any change in the level of advertising are based upon estimates from the observed data variations. Advertising expenditures do not vary that much from year to year so that estimating the effect of zero expenditure is well outside the normal range of prediction. It could also be hypothesized that an advertising ban, or any new advertising restriction, might have additional effects over a substantial reduction in expenditure. Such a ban may reinforce health education efforts and be seen as a clear statement of the Government's position on the harmful effects of smoking or alcohol misuse.

To overcome some of these problems other studies have used natural experiments of changes in legislation or pooled data across countries with different advertising restrictions (Cox and Smith 1984; Smart 1988; Laugesen and Meads 1991; Saffer 1991). Specific country studies of legislation changes have been difficult to interpret because of cross-border effects and industry lobbying (Smart and Cutler 1976). It is also important to separate out the effect of advertising restrictions from other effects. In the USA the television advertising ban was accompanied by a large drop in health education messages, and both Hamilton (1972) and Schneider *et al.* (1981) found that the health scare advertisements had been more effective in reducing consumption than advertising had been in increasing consumption.

Data pooled across countries may help to avoid some of these problems. Cox and Smith (1984) estimated separate demand functions for tobacco over a number of countries. The effect of the unobservable advertising policy variables were hypothesized to affect coefficient estimates. More restrictive advertising policy was found to decrease consumption, but only 2 of the 15 countries had well-established legislative policies. Another problem with this study was that it may be expected that coefficient estimates would be different before and after major policy changes as well as between studies.

Structural stability within countries was also assumed by Laugesen and Meads (1991). Data from OECD countries were pooled for the years 1960–1986. An alcohol advertising restriction score was calculated which could take a value between 0 and 1 for each country in each year. This score as found to be inversely related to consumption. The construction and use of this score would lead to the assumption that a score of 10 would have twice the effect on consumption as a score of 5. This is a restrictive model and it would have been useful to test other specifications of the advertising restriction term.

Saffer (1991) found that broadcast alcohol advertising bans reduced consumption. In this study the relationship between alcohol consumption, liver cirrhosis, motor vehicle fatalities, and advertising was analysed with a pooled time-series for 17 countries. An 'alcohol sentiment' variable was included to avoid the possibility of spurious relationships between advertising bans and consumption. The author concludes that the empirical results support the view that the countries with broadcast advertising bans have lower levels of alcohol consumption and other measures of alcohol misuse.

Availability

Both alcohol and tobacco sales are subject to a number of restrictions which may be expected to have an effect on the demand and the supply of the products. The effect of regulations and how they interact with economic factors have been studied for alcohol but not generally for tobacco (Godfrey 1986a). Specific effects considered in alcohol studies include the number and type of outlet (McGuinness 1983; Godfrey 1988), the effects of state monopolies (Ornstein and Hanssens 1985; Holder and Wagenaar 1990), and the effect of strikes (Osterberg and Saila 1991). These studies suggest that relaxation in alcohol availability leads to some overall increase in alcohol consumption, although the effects vary across beverages. In addition, data from natural experiments in Finland caused by strikes suggest that 'aggregate alcohol consumption and consumption of frequently drinking groups and alcohol abusers as well as adverse consequences of alcohol can be affected by controlling the alcohol availability' (Osterberg and Saila 1991).

Health information

The impact of the considerable publicity about the dangers of smoking have been incorporated in economic models in different ways (Godfrey 1986a). The effects have included estimates of the immediate effects on consumption of a 'health shock' and whether the effects of these shocks fade or continue. For example, one estimate of UK cigarette consumption suggests that there were immediate falls in consumption at the times of major publicity about the effects of smoking and a continual effect resulting in a fall of consumption of about 3 per cent a year (Godfrey and Maynard 1988). Schneider *et al.* (1981) extended the analysis of health education effects to include changes in the type of cigarette consumed.

Most empirical studies have concluded that health publicity has decreased cigarette demand, but the measures used to estimate these effects are crude and it is difficult to extrapolate these results to future events. Two recent studies have examined these effects in a different way (Tegene 1991; Seldon and Boyd 1991). Although they used different methods in both studies it was assumed that health information events would affect the stability of the demand model and all the parameter estimates. Both did find structural breaks around health events, but the studies differed in the estimates of the significance of later events and advertising parameters.

Models linking economic factors, consumption levels, and abuse

One of the major problems of using population estimates of how changes in economic factors change consumption is that these consumption changes may not be necessarily directly linked to changes in drug-related problems. There have been a number of attempts to link models of alcohol consumption and problems. Schweitzer *et al.* (1983) estimated a system of equations for the joint determination of alcohol consumption, alcoholism, and alcohol-related mortality. Maynard (1983) criticized elements of the model which could invalidate the presented results, but further development of the model could be both interesting and informative to policy makers.

There is a much wider body of literature on the effects of both tax and specific measures on drink-driving fatalities (Tether and Godfrey 1990). Saffer and Grossman (1987) allowed for the possibility that not only could drinking-age laws affect consumption, but also that changes in the law may be influenced by levels of consumption via an impact on drink-driving mortalities. The importance of including these sentiment effects and allowing for the possibility of feedback between variables has been considered in a number of studies. Results show that ignoring these type of effects can lead to misleading results. In a later study Chaloupka *et al.* (1991) investigated the effectiveness of a wide range of measures which may affect both youth and all age driving mortality rates in the USA. They concluded that the most effective policies are increased beer taxes and mandatory administrative license actions. Maintaining the beer tax at its real 1951 value would have reduced fatalities by 11.5 per cent annually during the period 1982–1988.

Summary

The empirical studies suggest that prices and income are important factors in determining changes in population levels of substance use. Estimates of the importance of these economic factors vary between substances, across countries, and with economic circumstances. The effect of advertising has been particularly difficult to estimate, but this may change as data become available from countries who have imposed complete tobacco advertising bans. A small but growing number of studies also suggests a direct relationship between economic factors and indicators of alcohol misuse, with studies of road traffic fatalities beginning to give some policy guidance on the effectiveness of tax compared to more specific measures.

ECONOMIC FACTORS AND INDIVIDUAL SUBSTANCE USE

Population level studies cannot be expected to provide much evidence about the comparative strengths of economic, cultural, and social factors in determining substance use. Some studies using data pooled across time and states have included variables to measure effects such as religion, unemployment rates, ethnic group, gender, and age, but few dominant patterns emerge (Godfrey 1986a; Ponicki 1990).

As well as the interactions between social and economic factors it would also be useful to investigate whether the nature and size of relationships varied between groups of the population. Some groups will be of particular policy interest. For example, if heavy drinkers respond to price changes with smaller consumption changes than other drinkers, then a tax increase will be a less effective means of reducing alcohol-related problems than an overall population estimate would predict.

Rather than using survey data to estimate these type of effects, Cook and Tauchen (1982) used cirrhosis mortality rates as a proxy for heavy drinking and examined how economic factors influences these rates. Using a pooled time-series across USA states they concluded that heavy drinkers were responsive to price changes. Kendell *et al.* (1983) also found evidence to support the view that heavy drinkers reduce consumption if prices rise. Using survey data collected before and after a large tax increase, they concluded that heavy drinkers and dependent drinkers in Scotland reduced their consumption at least as much as light and moderate drinkers. Townsend (1987), using survey data on smoking aggregated over social groups, found some evidence that there may be a gradient in the price elasticity estimates, with men in the lowest social groups being more price responsive than those in the higher groups. These results were, however, based on parameter estimates that were not statistically significant.

There are problems with using survey data. Grossing up estimates from regular household surveys suggest that consumption is seriously underestimated when compared to the time-series data. The shortfall from UK surveys has, for example, been estimated at 22–26 per cent for tobacco and 40–45 per cent for alcohol (Kemsley *et al.* 1980). One reason for these discrepancies is that heavy drinkers and smokers may be less likely to be included in the sample design and more likely to be non-respondents. While these regular surveys provide a rich micro-data set, care is needed in interpreting results.

Detailed analysis of household expenditure patterns have been undertaken both in the UK and the USA (Heien and Pompelli 1989; Atkinson *et al.* 1989; Baker and McKay 1990). The results for UK data suggest considerable variations of income elasticities with income and characteristics such as age, occupation, and sex composition of households for alcohol. The model described in Baker and McKay (1990) is interesting in that demand is estimated separately for four separate groups, divided into smoking and car ownership status. Beer price elasticities show considerable variations across these groups with an estimate of −1.27 for the non-car but smoker households to −0.36 for the car owner but non-smoker households. There are, however, considerable difficulties in obtaining precise price elasticity estimates from these analyses of household data (Atkinson *et al.* 1989). The results from the USA study yield negative income coefficients, but the data were restricted to alcohol consumed in the home (Heien and Pompelli 1989).

Analysis of tobacco expenditure patterns have taken a different form with more complex specifications of demand, to take account of the number of households with no tobacco expenditure. This leads to separate participation and consumption equations. Another interesting use of these household data is the construction of a pseudo cohort to study patterns of consumption over the lifecycle (Browning 1987). He found that the presence of young children did not reduce the consumption of tobacco significantly and reduced consumption of alcohol only a little.

Despite the richness of these data sets there are problems in interpreting results for health policy purposes. Household behaviour is an aggregation over different numbers in each household and types of individuals. For a household to be classed as non-smoking, for example, all members of that household have to be non-smokers, and trends in this variable may be very different than trends in overall smoking participation. Also some results are difficult to explain. Owner occupation has been found to be a significant determinant in some studies, but this variable could be acting as a proxy for a number of socio-economic characteristics.

There are a number of studies using individual data. Lewit *et al.* (1981) studied the smoking habits of teenagers, and their results suggested that this group were more responsive to both price and health education messages than estimates obtained from aggregate studies had indicated. Price elasticities of smoking prevalence were also found to be much larger that the price elasticity of quantity smoked.

A more recent study has examined how excise taxes and smoking regulation affect individual smoking behaviour (Wasserman *et al.* 1991).

A regulation score was used which could take four values between 0 and 1. The estimates of price effects were found to be lower that in other American studies based on individual data. Grossman (1991) comments that the results were sensitive to the inclusion of the regulation index and that the relationship between the index and smoking sentiment in the area had not been examined. These results are interesting, however, and the effect of smoking restriction in workplaces and public places merits further research.

Surveys which could examine changing substance misuse habits would be of particular interest. For example, it would be useful to know whether a substantial tax increase for cigarettes had larger effects on quitting than would be predicted from the application of simple price elasticities. Jones (1989*b*) has proposed and tested a model which looked at participation, quitting, and tobacco consumption. This study was conducted with only a single year of UK survey data and, therefore, it was not possible to estimate price effects, but it would be useful to extend this type of analysis to a pooled series.

There have also been a number of American studies looking at the effects of economic factors on individual alcohol consumption (as reviewed by Grossman 1989). Their results on the effectiveness of both minimum drinking-age laws and beer taxes are similar to those described above on population data.

To summarize, the number of studies investigating the effect of economic factors on different groups of the population or individuals' substance misuse have been far fewer than the population studies. Evidence does suggest that coefficient estimates will vary but that both light and heavy consumers are likely to be affected by changes in economic factors.

ECONOMIC THEORIES OF DEPENDENCE AND ADDICTION

Many of the economic studies of the factors influencing the consumption of alcohol and tobacco have made no allowance for any dependence, habit, or addiction. There has, however, been a growing interest in developing models linking economic and social behaviour theories. One way that economists have attempted to make some allowance for dependence is to include a term for past consumption in population studies (Godfrey 1986*a*). Different models specified the effect as a stock, as measuring an adjustment process, or simply including past consumption as a proxy for habit.

While habit models may capture some notion of tolerance, they do not incorporate other potential features of addictive demand. By examining the process by which individuals make choices some economists have attempted to explain behaviour with models which may lead to harm but in which individuals still act rationally to maximize their own welfare. Birch and Stoddart (1990) outlined a taxonomy of the different factors influencing individuals' choice of harmful behaviours. Attitudes towards risk and time preference rates were two of the factors identified. Different rates of valuing future health benefits from changes in smoking behaviour, that is different time preference rates, have been found to be related to educational attainment among the young (Farrell and Fuchs 1982). Hence, dependence could result from rational consumption over time when individuals choose to place a high weight on the benefits of current consumption (avoidance of withdrawal costs) and a low weight on future costs (health and social problems). In these circumstances it may be rational to demand policies, such as taxes, to help change behaviour (Crain *et al.* 1977).

More specific addiction models have been developed and tested with cigarette consumption data. As well as dependence, the model tested by Young (1983) includes a type of withdrawal effect. In this model it is assumed that some degree of addiction may result in consumers responding asymmetrically to changes in economic factors. In particular, consumers may have a tendency to acquire a habit more easily at times of low prices or high income and then may be reluctant to abandon the habit if prices rise or incomes fall. This has important policy implications because, if such asymmetries exist, policies to restore tax levels to some previous real level would not be sufficient to reduce consumption levels to the original level, even if all other factors remain constant. Real tax levels are often allowed to fall in real terms over substantial periods of time.

Young (1983) evaluated this model using US data and found asymmetric price effects. Instead of an estimate that would suggest that a price rise of 10 per cent would lower consumption by 4.5 per cent, the asymmetric price results suggest that a rise in prices of 14 per cent would be required to achieve the same 4.5 per cent reduction in consumption. This model has also been evaluated for the UK (Godfrey and Maynard 1988) and Finland (Pekurinen 1989). In the Finnish study the demand for cigarettes was found to be twice as sensitive to falling prices (-0.94) than to rising prices (-0.49). This study was also unusual in that cross-price effects for tobacco products were studied. Less support for the Young model was found when applied to UK data.

The Young model has been specified and tested with population data. Other addiction models have been developed for use with individual data. For example, Jones (1988) developed a model for tobacco demand incorporating both asymmetries of demand and a measure of social interaction between smokers and non-smokers.

The most extensive economic model of rational addiction has been proposed by Becker and Murphy (1988). In their theoretical model, addicts are assumed to be rational in that they are forward looking and maximize their utility or satisfaction from consumption over time. This is in contrast to the Young model where consumers are assumed to be myopic. In the Becker and Murphy model an individual's well being at any moment is assumed to depend on health, the psychological and physiological benefits of consuming the addictive substance and the benefits derived from the consumption of all other goods. Health is expected to depend, amongst other things, on the cumulative past consumption of the addictive substance, that is the addictive 'stock'. The benefits of current consumption of the addictive substance are assumed to depend on current levels of use and the addictive stock. Greater past consumption is predicted to have a negative effect on the benefits gained from current consumption, that is there is a tolerance effect. Withdrawal effects are captured by assuming total utility falls if consumption of the addictive substance is reduced. Reinforcement effects are allowed for by the assumption that the extra utility or benefit gained from a small increase in current consumption is larger as past consumption is greater, that is past consumption reinforces current consumption.

The mathematical model proposed by Becker and Murphy yields a number of interesting predictions. For example, permanent changes in prices may have small short-run effects, but the long-run demand for addictive goods is predicted to be more elastic than the demand for non-addictive goods. Some addictive behaviour patterns, such as 'binges', abrupt discontinuity of consumption, and repeated quitting behaviour are also consistent with this model of 'rational' behaviour.

The demand equation derived from the theory includes future and past price and consumption terms. The significance of these terms gives a test of the consistency of the theory with the data. There have been a number of attempts to test this model with both population and individual data. Becker *et al.* (1987), using a time series of state cross-sections for cigarette consumption, found support for the theory with the long-run price elasticity estimate of -0.77 being considerably higher than the short-run estimate of -0.44. Chaloupka (1991) applied the model to individual data and also found support for the rational addiction theory of smoking behaviour. In comparing across age and educational attainment, he concluded that less educated and younger individuals were found to behave more myopically than the more educated and older individuals. There was also evidence to support the hypothesis that the more addicted individuals will be more responsive in the long run to changes in price than less addicted individuals.

Development of economic models of addictive behaviour are much newer and relatively untested compared to other behavioural sciences, but they do provide an interesting starting point for a more comprehensive examination of the role of economic factors.

SUPPLIERS AND THEIR EFFECTS ON ADDICTION MARKETS

The main focus of this paper has been on how economic factors may influence the decisions of consumers of different substances. However, both the goods offered, that is the availability of less dangerous goods, and their prices are influenced by the behaviour of producers, distributers, and retailers. If markets are very competitive, then economic theory would suggest that market forces would ensure efficiency among firms and that no supplier would have sufficient power to influence the market. In reality, both the alcohol and tobacco markets bear little resemblance to the economic benchmark model. Both tobacco companies and brewers tend to be large companies and sometimes multinational. Concern has been expressed about the behaviour of both tobacco and alcohol companies in developing countries.

In the UK, both the alcohol and tobacco markets are dominated by a few firms (Booth *et al.* 1990). Economic theory suggests that in such markets firms will not compete through price but through other forms of competition, such as advertising and brand proliferation, and these characteristics may be seen in the alcohol and tobacco industries.

The tobacco and alcohol industries also have a long history of regulation in the UK which creates a network of interdependence between government, bureaucrats, and industry. Producer groups will lobby to seek to minimize the impact of any potential restrictive policy and firms will act to neutralize the actual effects of current policy. The tobacco industry, for example, reacted to advertising restrictions by competitions, then by sponsoring sports and other events, followed by marketing strategies which put logos on clothes and other goods, and more recently by financing retail shops to have prominent signs. Producers will campaign vigorously against certain measures and seek to influence debate with alarmist forecasts of the effects of policy change. The tobacco industry have, for example, run a number of campaigns before Budgets warning of job losses and increased imports if taxes are raised (Leedham and Godfrey, 1990). Evidence about the effectiveness of these lobbying activities are, however, mixed and may vary considerably across different issues (Godfrey and Powell, 1991).

Although industry lobbies are generally seen to be more cohesive than health and social groups, interests among producers, distributers, and retailers will not always coincide. In particular, reforms to the brewing industry and license laws in the UK have seen some divisions between brewers, supermarket chains, and public house tenants. Also, the spirits industry has long campaigned to have tax per unit alcohol equalized between beverages. Health lobbies and trade lobbies may not always disagree over policy changes although their reasons for support or opposition may differ. For example, increasing competition from deregulation in an industry may lead to losses for existing firms and if price competition increases, the resulting fall in price may increase consumption leading to an increase in health and social problems.

Some prevention policies may have unexpected consequences. If advertising is banned, for example, firms may not only reduce costs but use price competition rather than advertising to compete for consumers. To fully evaluate all policy changes it is necessary to examine all possible changes in both consumers and producers behaviour.

The influence of supply on legal drug use has largely been ignored. For illicit drugs, in contrast, considerable resources are spent attempting to influence supply. Drug markets are complicated with many stages between the producer and sale to a user and, therefore plenty of different levels where law enforcement effort can be directed. Wagstaff and Maynard (1988) examined the cost-effectiveness of different law enforcement activities in the UK. Data were too poor for definitive results. Careful economic analysis of markets do yield the conclusion that *a priori* no conclusions can be reached on where the most law enforcement resources should be deployed. While economic analysis has some uses in analysing supply and demand for illicit substances further work is hindered by a lack of data. Such data are only likely to be generated in collaborative projects.

CONCLUSIONS

There is a considerable body of economic research on the factors influencing alcohol and tobacco use at a population level. These analyses have been used in policy debates, but not always critically or constructively. Studies generally confirm that economic factors will have an important part in the process of changing population habits. For some factors, such as prices and advertising, policies are available which can influence changes in substance use. For other factors, such as income, changes are outside the control of those seeking to moderate harmful consequences of substance use and at some periods may mitigate their efforts.

The economists' contribution to the debate about controlling legal and illegal substance use has been largely empirical rather than theoretical. Increasing use of individual data and the development and testing of more specific addiction models may, however, bring economists more into the mainstream of addiction research.

There is a large research agenda. Few estimates are available of the variation of the effects of economic factors across different groups of the population. Further investigation of the young, different social groups, and the heavier consumers may be the most obvious priorities. Considerably more analyses of illicit drug markets are required.

The review of available studies suggest that markets and individuals are dynamic and that the influence of prices, incomes, and other economic factors will vary with time, prosperity, and changing social and cultural factors. Studies will vary in the estimates they produce. Care is needed in interpreting any empirical results. More rigorous statistical testing of models and more comparisons of competing theories would help debates, about how economic factors can be manipulated to affect change, to be constructively conducted.

REFERENCES

Ahtola, J., Ekholm, A., and Somervuori, A. (1986). Bayes estimates for the price and income elasticities of alcoholic beverages in Finland from 1955 to 1980. *Journal of Business and Economic Statistics*, **4**, 119–208.

Atkinson, A., Gomulka, J., nd Stern, N. (1989). Spending on beer, wine and spirits: evidence from the Family Expenditure Survey 1970–1983. *Discussion Paper 114, ESRC programme on taxation, incentives and the distribution of income*. London School of Economics, London.

Baker, P. and McKay, S. (1990). The structure of alcohol taxes: a hangover from the past? *IFS Commentary 21*. Institute for Fiscal Studies, London.

Becker, G. S. and Murphy, K. M. (1988). A theory of rational addiction. *Journal of Political Economy*, **96**, 675–700.

Becker, G. S., Grossman, M., and Murphy, K. M. (1987). An empirical analysis of cigarette addiction. *Working Paper*. Department of Economics, University of Chicago.

Birch, S. and Stoddart, G. (1990). Promoting healthy behaviour: the importance of economic analysis in policy formulation for AIDS prevention. *Health Policy*, **16**, 187–97.

Booth, M., Hartley, K., and Powell, M. (1990). Industry: structure, performance and policy. In *Preventing alcohol and tobacco problems*, Vol. 1 (ed. A. Maynard and P. Tether), pp. 151–78. Avebury, Aldershot.

Browning, M. (1987). Eating, drinking, smoking, and testing the lifecycle hypothesis. *The Quarterly Journal of Economics*, May, 329–45.

Chaloupka, F. (1991). Rational addictive behaviour and cigarette smoking. *Journal of Political Economy*, **99**, 722–42.

Chaloupka, F. J., Saffer, H., and Grossman M. (1991). Alcohol control policies and motor vehicle fatalities. *NBER Working Paper 3831*. NBER, Cambridge, Massachusetts.

Chetwynd, J., Coope, P., Brodie, R. J., and Wells, E. (1988). Impact of cigarette advertising on aggregate demand for cigarettes in New Zealand. *British Journal of Addiction*, **83**, 401–14.

Clements, K. W. and Johnson, L. W. (1983). The demand for beer, wine and spirits: a systemwide analysis. *Journal of Business*, **56**, 273–304.

Crain, M., Deaton, T., Holcombe, R. and Tollisons, R. (1977). Rational choice and the taxation of sin. *Journal of Public Economics*, **8**, 239–45.

Cook, P. J. and Tauchen, G. (1982). The effect of liquor taxes on heavy drinking. *Bell Journal of Economics*, **13**, 379–90.

Cox, H. and Smith, R. (1984). Political approaches to smoking control: a comparative analysis. *Applied Economics*, **16**, 569–82.

Duffy, M. H. (1987). Advertising and the inter-product distribution of demand: a Rotterdam model approach. *European Economic Review*, **31**, 1051–70.

Farrell, P. and Fuchs, V. R. (1982). Schooling and health: the cigarette connection. *Journal of Health Economics*, **1**, 217–30.

Glen, D. and Carr-Hill, J. (1991). Modelling the demand for alcoholic drinks: a cointegrated approach. *Working Papers in Economics 9*. Polytechnic of West London, London.

Godfrey, C. (1986*a*). Factors influencing the consumption of alcohol and tobacco: a review of demand models. *Discussion Paper 17*. Centre for Health Economics, University of York.

Godfrey, C. (1986*b*). Government policy, advertising and tobacco consumption in the UK: a critical review of the literature. *British Journal of Addiction*, **81**, 339–46.

Godfrey, C. (1988). Licensing and the demand for alcohol. *Applied Economics*, **20**, 1541–58.

Godfrey, C. (1989). Factors influencing the consumption of alcohol and tobacco: the use and abuse of economic models. *British Journal of Addiction*, **84**, 1123–38.

Godfrey, C. and Harrison, L. (1990) . In *Controlling alcohol and tobacco problems*, Vol. 1 (ed. A. Maynard and P. Tether), pp. 54–74. Avebury, Aldershot.

Godfrey, C. and Maynard, A. (1988). Economic aspects of tobacco use and taxation policy. *British Medical Journal*, **297**, 339–43.

Godfrey, C. and Posnett, J. (1988). An analysis of the distributional impact of taxes on alcohol and tobacco. *Working Paper*. Centre for Health Economics, University of York.

Godfrey, C. and Powell, M. (1991). Regulating addictive commodities: dependence and the culture of enterprise. In *Dependency to enterprise*, (ed. J. Hutton, S. Hutton, T. Pinch and A. Shiell), pp. 49–62. Routledge, London.

Grossman, M. (1989). Health benefits of increases in alcohol and cigarette taxes. *British Journal of Addiction*, **84**, 1193–204.

Grossman, M. (1991). The demand for cigarettes. *Journal of Health Economics*, **10**, 101–3.

Hamilton, J. L. (1972). The demand for cigarettes: advertising, the health scare and the cigarette advertising ban. *Review of Economics and Statistics*, **56**, 401–11.

Heien, D. and Pompelli, G. (1989). The demand for alcoholic beverages: economic and demographic effects. *Southern Economic Journal*, **55**, 759–70.

Holder, H. D. and Wagenaar, A. C. (1990). Effects of the elimination of a state monopoly on distilled spirits' retail sales: a time series analysis of Iowa. *British Journal of Addiction*, **85**, 1615–25.

Jones, A. (1988). Starters, quitters, and smokers: a microeconomic analysis of individuals' cigarette consumption. Paper presented to the health Economists' Study Group, University of Newcastle-upon-Tyne.

Jones, A. (1989*a*). A systems approach to the demand for alcohol and tobacco. *Bulletin of Economic Research*, **41**, 86–105.

Jones, A. (1989*b*). A double-hurdle model of cigarette consumption. *Journal of Applied Econometrics*, **4**, 23–39.

Kemsley, W. F. F., Redpath, R. U., and Holmes, M. (1980). *Family expenditure survey handbook*. HMSO, London.

Kendell, R. E., de Roumanie, M., and Ritson, E. B. (1983). Effects of economic change on Scottish drinking habits 1978–82. *British Journal of Addiction*, **78**, 365–79.

Laugesen, M. and Meads, C. (1991). Tobacco advertising restrictions, price, income and tobacco consumption in OECD countries, 1960–1986. *British Journal of Addiction*, **86**, 1343–54.

Leedham, W. and Godfrey, C. (1990). Tax policy and budget decisions. In *Preventing alcohol and tobacco problems*, Volume 1 (ed. A. Maynard and P. Tether), pp. 96–116. Avebury, Aldershot.

Lewit, E. M. (1989). U.S. tobacco taxes: behavioural effects and policy implications. *British Journal of Addiction*, **84**, 1217–34.

Lewit, E. M., Coate, D., and Grossman, M. (1981). The effects of government regulation on teenage smoking. *Journal of Law and Economics*, **25**, 545–69.

McGuinness, T. (1983). The demand for beer, spirits and wine in the UK, 1956–1975. In *Economics and alcohol* (ed. M. Grant, M. Plant, and A. Williams), pp. 238–42. Croom Helm, London.

Maynard, A. (1983). Modelling alcohol consumption and abuse: the power and pitfalls of economic techniques. In *Economics and alcohol* (ed. M. Grant, M. Plant, and A. Williams), pp. 128–39. Croom Helm, London.

Nisbet, C. T. and Vakil, F. (1972). Some estimates of price and expenditure elasticities of demand for marijuana among U.C.L.A. students. *The Review of Economics and Statistics*, **LIV**, pp. 473–5.

Ornstein, S.I. and Hanssens, D. M. (1985). Alcohol control laws and the consumption of distilled spirits and beer. *Journal of Consumer Research*, **12**, 200–13.

Osterberg, E. (1991). Current approaches to limit alcohol abuse and the negative consequences of use: a comparative overview of available options and an assessment of proven effectiveness. In *The negative social consequences of alcohol use* (ed. O. G. Aasland), pp. 266–93. Norwegian Ministry of Health and Social Affairs and the United Nations Office at Vienna Centre for Social Development and Humanitarian Affairs, Oslo.

Osterberg, E. and Saila, S-L. (ed.) (1991). *Natural experiments with decreased availability of alcohol beverages. Finnish alcohol strikes in 1972 and 1985.* The Finnish Foundation for Alcohol Studies, Helsinki.

Pekurinen, M. (1989). The demand for tobacco products in Finland. *British Journal of Addiction*, **84**, 1183–92.

Ponicki, W. (1990). The price and income elasticities of the demand for alcohol: a review of the literature. *Working Paper*. Prevention Research Center, Berkeley.

Powell, M. (1989). Alcohol and tobacco tax harmonisation in the European Community. In *Controlling legal addictions* (ed. D. Robinson, A. Maynard and R. Chester), pp. 131–47. Macmillan, London.

Saffer, H. (1991). Alcohol advertising bans and alcohol abuse: an international perspective. *Journal of Health Economics*, **10**, 65–79.

Saffer, H. and Grossman, M. (1987). Drinking age laws and highway mortality rate: cause and effect. *Economic Inquiry*, **25**, 403–77.

Salvananthan, E. A. (1988). The demand for alcohol in the UK: an economic study. *Applied Economics*, **20**, 1071–86.

Schneider, L., Klein, B., and Murphy, K. M. (1981). Government regulation of cigarette health information. *Journal of Law and Economics*, **24**, 575–612.

Schweitzer, S. O., Intriligator, M. D., and Salehi, J. (1983). In *Economics and alcohol* (ed. M. Grant, M. Plant, and A. Williams), pp. 107–27. Croom Helm, London.

Seldon, B. J. and Boyd, R. (1991). The stability of cigarette demand. *Applied Economics*, **23**, 319–26.

Silverman, L. P. and Spruill, N. L. (1977). Urban crime and the price of heroin. *Journal of Urban Economics*, **4**, 80–103.

Smart, R. G. (1988). Does alcohol advertising affect overall consumption? A review of empirical studies. *Journal of Studies on Alcohol*, **49**, 314–23.

Smart, R. G. and Cutler, R. E. (1976). The alcohol advertising ban in British Columbia: problems and effects on beverage consumption. *British Journal of Addiction*, **71**, 13–21.

Sparrow, M., Brazeau, R., Collins, H., and Morrison, R. A. (1989). *Alcoholic beverage taxation and control policies*, 7th ed. Brewers Association of Canada, Ontario.

Tegene, A. (1991). Kalman filter and the demand for cigarettes. *Applied Economics*, **23**, 1175–82.

Tether, P. and Godfrey, C. (1990). Drinking and driving. In *Preventing alcohol and tobacco problems*, Vol. 2 (ed. C. Godfrey and D. Robinson), pp. 139–165. Avebury, Aldershot.

Townsend, J. (1987). Cigarette tax, economic welfare and social class patterns of smoking. *Applied Economics*, **19**, 355–65.

Wagstaff, A. (1989). Economic aspects of illicit drug markets and drug enforcement policies. *British Journal of Addiction*, **84**, 1173–82.

Wagstaff, A. and Maynard, A. (1988). *Economic aspects of the illicit drug market and drug enforcement policies in the United Kingdom.* HMSO, London.

Walsh, B. M. (1982). The demand for alcohol in the UK: a comment. *Journal of Industrial Economics,* **30,** 439–46.

Wasserman, J., Manning, W. G., Newhouse, J. P., and Winkler, J. D. (1991). The effects of excise taxes and regulations on cigarette smoking. *Journal of Health Economics,* **10,** 43–64.

Young, T. (1983). The demand for cigarettes: alternative specifications of Fujii's model. *Applied Economics,* **15,** 203–11.

10

Diffusion of innovation as a model for understanding population change in substance use

ROBERTA FERRENCE

INTRODUCTION

Psychoactive drugs are not typically thought of as innovations in the way that new technologies or inventions are. Yet, the introduction and spread of these substances in any society occur in much the same way as the adoption and diffusion of other new products and processes. My purpose in this chapter is to describe the ways in which changes in patterns of substance use fit the diffusion of innovation model, to provide examples of ways in which this model can illuminate our thinking about substance use, and to propose a research agenda based on this model. A number of examples are from smoking research, but I have included illustrations for all types of substance use.

Many theories of substance use explain behaviour in terms of individual factors, whether psychosocial, physiological, or genetic. Theories of cigarette smoking, for example, usually focus on the individual and often their pathology (Ashton and Stepney 1982), or are physiological, ascribing patterns of use to the addictive qualities of nicotine (Russell 1971). The small body of research that looks at group behaviour is largely economic, using changes in pricing and taxation to explain trends in smoking (Lewit and Coate 1982; Godfrey 1989). Yet, in none of this research do we find satisfying explanations for many changes in substance use patterns in the general population or in specific subgroups, such as women, young people, disadvantaged groups, and particular ethnic groups. For example, why was cigarette smoking in western cultures most prevalent among the highly educated early in this century, whereas it is now most common among the economically disadvantaged? Some current thought on smoking suggests that powerlessness contributes to smoking and that women and those with low incomes smoke because they lack control. One is left to wonder why the first smokers were from among the elite, who were certainly neither powerless nor lacking in control. Similar changes can be seen for other substances, such as alcohol use and illicit drug use, and for other variables, such as age, sex, and geographic location. Individual-focused theories and macro-level economic theories are certainly useful in explaining some of the variation in substance-use behaviour. Yet, none of them fully satisfy our curiosity about the ebb and flow of levels of use and the convergences and divergences among different groups.

DIFFUSION OF INNOVATION MODELS

What is the 'diffusion of innovation' and why might we be interested in applying it to substance use? Diffusion of innovation refers to the spread of new ideas, techniques, behaviour, or products throughout a population. The cumulative rate of adoption of innovations is characterized by an S-shaped curve which increases slowly at first, then more rapidly, and finally slows and levels off. In some cases, there is a decline or discontinuance, which follows much the same pattern as the increase (Fig. 10.1).

Early work by Gabriel Tarde (1903) described diffusion as a form of imitation which filtered down from higher to lower socioeconomic levels. He also suggested that imitation was a function of proximity, with the fastest spread occurring in areas with the highest density. These concepts were later incorporated in more detailed models, most

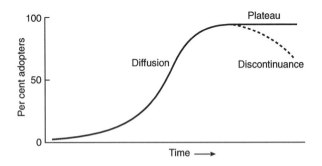

FIG. 10.1 Diffusion curve for adoption of innovation.

importantly by Rogers and Shoemaker (1971, 1983), but also by Barnett (1953), Griliches (1957), Brown (1981), and many others.

Davis (1985) describes three perspectives that involve models used in diffusion theory. The *rational/economic* perspective includes both *economic* and *structural* models. These are generally applied to explain the diffusion of new products or processes in terms of economic and structural variables, including size of company and factors related to the investment of resources and structural characteristics of the companies. While structural factors are more relevant to organizations than individuals, and since substance use tends to spread among individuals, the diffusion of licit drugs, for example, would undoubtedly be related to structural factors in the medical profession, pharmaceutical industry, and government. These might include the influence of medical associations, the degree of competition within the industry, and whether or not the responsibility for regulation of pharmaceuticals is located within a health ministry or one concerned with commercial relations. Similarly, the spread of illicit drugs would depend on the structure of the illicit market.

The *economic* model would clearly be relevant at both the organizational and individual level. Economic factors in the production and distribution of cocaine, for example, would determine supply and pricing to individual users, and individual resources would also influence consumption. Add to this what might be called the cost−benefit aspects of using an illicit substance. Economic and personal benefits of sale and use need to be weighed against the likelihood of a distributor or user getting caught and the potential adverse effects, such as fines, incarcerations, and damage to reputation and employment prospects.

The *behavioural* perspective includes both *communications* and *champion* models. Rogers and Shoemaker (1983) emphasize the communication aspect of diffusion in their work. The mechanism for diffusion of innovations is communication, whether interpersonal or through media or other channels. The speed of adoption of any innovation relates to its source, its characteristics, the channels of communication available, and the characteristics of the adopters. The more credible and respected the source, the greater the likelihood of adoption. The relative advantage of a new product over existing alternatives, its compatibility with existing values, its complexity (or conversely, ease of understanding and use), the risk involved in trying it out (trialability), and the ease with which its use can be observed (observability) all affect the rate of adoption. Channels of communication, whether mass media, targeted interventions, or word of mouth, are critical components of the diffusion process.

Finally, adopters can be categorized on the basis of when they adopt innovations. Rogers has categorized them as innovators, early adopters, early or late majority adopters, and laggards, depending on how early or late they adopt.

The *champion* model focuses on the role of the innovator in organizations. Those with the greatest access to sources of communication and with the greatest orientation outside their own group tend to lead in the adoption of innovations. In general, males, those with higher socioeconomic status, especially education, those with status aspirations, those with greater access to sources of communication, and residents of large urban communities tend to be innovators or early adopters. In the substance-use area, these characteristics would characterize those most likely to adopt new substances when they appear in retail outlets (for example, low-alcohol beer) or through illicit channels (for example, cocaine). However, when the sources of new products are more specialized, such as physicians, who control access to new prescription drugs, early adopters would tend to be those who visit physicians most often, namely women and the elderly. In this case, characteristics of the prescribing physician, rather than the patient, might be more important in predicting prescription drug use.

The discontinuance phase follows much the same pattern as the diffusion phase. In fact, this phase can be viewed as the adoption of non-use. Early quitters also have the same characteristics as early adopters. For example, the first smokers to give up tobacco for health reasons were well-educated, urban males. This group had greater access to sources of information about the hazards of smoking, such as the 1964 Surgeon General's Report, and would be more likely to know others who had suffered from smoking-related diseases, because this was the group who adopted smoking first (Ferrence 1989). Even the nature of the evidence supported early discontinuance by this group. The first major published study on lung cancer was carried out on British doctors (Doll and Hill 1954).

Just as new substances may replace more benign products in the adoption phase, discontinuance may involve the adoption of non-psychoactive replacements. For example, beer drinkers may switch to de-alcoholized beer; wine drinkers may substitute mineral water on some occasions; and former smokers may switch to chewing gum. Research on the diffusion and discontinuance of different substances should also consider the role of replacements and determine the extent to which psychoactive and non-psychoactive products substitute for each other or are simply added to existing levels of use.

The *systems* perspective (Davis 1985) includes both a *marketing* and a *contextual* model. The *marketing* model attempts to incorporate entrepreneurial factors that affect adoption behaviour. These include number of outlets, pricing policy, promotional activity aimed at particular

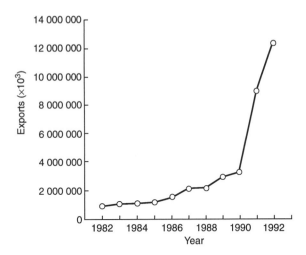

FIG. 10.2 Exports of Canadian cigarettes, 1982–92.

groups, and market segmentation. For example, while young people are influenced to use tobacco by their friends and family, the availability of tobacco to underage youth in neighbourhood outlets, the advertising and promotion of new and existing tobacco products, and the availability of small packages aimed at young people, are critical factors in the rate and extent of adoption, independent of interpersonal factors. The importance of these factors can be seen in the marketing failure of new tobacco products aimed at the youth market in Canada, where tobacco advertising has been banned since 1988. Current efforts to require licensing of tobacco outlets, with fines and licence revocation for sales to minors, can be seen as efforts to slow the adoption of cigarette smoking among future cohorts of young people. However, the continued profitability of the tobacco industry encourages the development of alternative marketing strategies. Since the Canadian advertising ban on tobacco was implemented, investment in promotion and sponsorship has grown dramatically.

The *contextual* model involves factors that 'are external to the innovating organization, but ... affect intraorganizational processes' (Tornatzky *et al.* 1983; Davis, 1985). These include interorganizational relationships and government policies. In Canada, the smuggling of exported cigarettes back into the country, which has increased exponentially in the past few years, provides a clear example of the contextual model. Lower cigarette taxes in the United States mean that Canadian cigarettes exported legally to the USA and smuggled back into Canada, can be sold at much lower prices than those sold legally in Canada. (Fig. 10.2 shows the diffusion of exports to the USA since 1982. While some of the cigarettes are purchased legally in the USA, mostly by Canadian visitors, there is no evidence that the legal market has increased significantly in recent years, so that most of the increase reflects smuggling.) The availability of a tax-exempt conduit back to Canada through Native reserves, combined with the large disparity in tax levels in the two countries, has led to the substantial illegal trade in Canadian cigarettes, now estimated at close to 40 per cent of total consumption. A short-lived export tax, which appeared to be effective in reducing smuggling, was removed after extensive lobbying by the industry. Voluntary reductions in exports on the part of one company were subsequently abandoned when other companies filled the gap and the 'complaint' company complained of unfair competition. While this has put considerable pressure on the government to reduce taxes, efforts in the USA to increase taxes to rates closer to those of Canada and western Europe and a reimposition of the export tax would eliminate much of the profit to be made and discontinue the diffusion of illicit cigarette use.

APPLICATIONS OF DIFFUSION MODELS

Specific studies of the diffusion of innovations include innovations as diverse as the adoption of hybrid corn (Griliches 1957), the use of credit cards (Malecki 1977), and the spread of collective violence (Pitcher *et al.* 1978). One of the first applications in the medical area involved a major study of the introduction of a new antibiotic (Coleman *et al.* 1966). A more recent study focused on the spread of surgical techniques (Sloan *et al.* 1986). A number of researchers have suggested that applying the model to substance use would be fruitful (Bell and Champion 1976; Blackford 1977; Robb 1986), yet, few have done so.

The application of diffusion theory to substance use has been largely in terms of an epidemic model. Epidemiologists have traditionally used an epidemic model, also characterized by an S-shaped curve, to study the spread of infectious diseases. The adoption of a new product or behaviour is analogous to contracting an infectious disease. Proponents of the innovation can be viewed as vectors or carriers. Techniques to prevent the adoption of substance use have been referred to as inoculation (Pfau *et al.* 1992). The best-known applications have been for substances that are often characterized as epidemic in their spread. Early work in the 1970s (Hughes and Crawford, 1972; Greene *et al.*

1974) typifies this approach. Greene and colleagues sought to test the 'ripple theory', which describes the spread of adoption of heroin use from large metropolitan areas with high density to smaller cities with lower population density and greater geographical isolation.

Musto (1989, 1992) describes the diffusion and decline of the first US cocaine epidemic, beginning in 1885 and lasting until the 1920s. Earlier, a wine containing coca-leaf extract, *Vin Mariani*, was developed and became widely admired, ultimately receiving a gold medal from the Pope. Commercial production of cocaine, beginning in the 1880s, was accompanied by extensive promotion by both drug companies and physicians, not only as a general tonic, but as the solution to hay fever (Musto, 1989). Its place as an ingredient in Coca Cola guaranteed it widespread diffusion throughout North America. By 1900, a variety of factors, including fear of violence associated with cocaine use, resulted in its withdrawal from medicinal uses and ultimately, severe restrictions on use. Subsequent increases and decreases in rates of cocaine use have occurred, but nothing as major as this first epidemic, when it changed from a much touted remedy to a widely feared drug in less than a generation.

This early cocaine epidemic invites comparison with the more recent rise and decline in cigarette smoking. Use of manufactured cigarettes did not become widespread in North America until World War I, when free cigarettes were distributed to troops in the field. Ease of use, great availability, and the close proximity of users led to rapid increases in rates of use during the 1920s, mainly among males. The massive entry of women into the labour force during World War II greatly accelerated their adoption of cigarette smoking. The publication in the 1950s of information about the health effects of smoking, followed by years of public education programmes, and restrictions on use, has resulted in a steady decline in the prevalence of smoking in most western countries. Unlike cocaine, which was largely wiped out by changes in its legal status and increased public fears as to its dangers, tobacco use continues to be widespread, although reduced, and tobacco remains a legal commodity.

APPLYING THE DIFFUSION MODEL IN ADDICTIONS RESEARCH

The limited use of diffusion theory in substance-use research belies its promise as a tool for mapping and explaining patterns and trends in different populations at different periods. What might be useful directions for diffusion research on addictions at this time?

There are two main ways in which the diffusion model can be applied to the study of population change in substance use: first, as a model for explaining patterns and trends in general populations and subpopulations, and second, as a way of identifying the most effective approaches to changing patterns of use.

The diffusion model is most useful for explaining existing trends, and possibly for predicting future trends. Researchers often assume a linear model for substance use, which is understandable when one looks at only a small part of the diffusion curve. However, attempting to predict long-term patterns on this basis can provide very misleading results. For example, the likelihood that substance use will ultimately fall to zero is very small. Yet, applying a linear model to a decline in substance use will produce that result.

Knowledge of the diffusion curve which is clearly non-linear, allows the researcher to expect a levelling off, that is not necessarily the result of flagging control measures. What it more likely describes is a point at which the remaining users are those least likely to be affected by social control and educational strategies—the heavily addicted and the socially marginal user. Or, it may result from a reduction in social concern, evidenced by fewer control measures and allocation of resources to prevention, as the size of the problem decreases.

Intervention efforts at this point may need to involve very different approaches. Plotting separate diffusion curves for particular groups may indicate that they are at a different point on the diffusion curve than the rest of the population. In Canada, for example, residents of Quebec have higher rates of smoking than residents of most other provinces. While efforts have been made to explain this in terms of cultural factors and differences in health attitudes relating to Franco-phones (Létourneau 1989), smoking actually rose more slowly in that province early in this century, and began to decline at a later date (Ferrence 1989). This may be due to the language barrier, reflected in both social networks and media influence, which prevented new behaviours from crossing into Quebec society. Current levels of smoking among Francophones are decreasing at rates similar to those of Anglophones (Ferrence and Kozlowski 1990), so the relevant question is not, why do Francophones smoke more than Anglophones, but where are they on the discontinuance curve, and what are the implications for future rates of smoking and problems.

A similar process has occurred with women, who began smoking in large numbers about twenty years after men did, suffered health effects later, were only included in epidemiological studies at a later point, and have only recently been determined to suffer the same health consequences as men (USHHS 1980). Despite the fact that smoking peaked and began to decline in the 1970s in the USA, for example, the belief prevails that smoking is still increasing among women.

Reference to the diffusion process can help clarify what has happened in the past and what is likely to occur in the future for a number of groups who adopted smoking or other substances at a later stage. It can temper conclusions based on linear models of change, and can provide a basis for looking beyond the characteristics of particular groups for the commonalities they share that affect the adoption process. Thus, we can expect that women, those with lower socioeconomic status, and those with more marginal status, such as Native Peoples, will be identified as difficult to educate because they discontinue use later than those who are more advantaged. Of course, their lesser access to sources of communication do make them harder to reach, but this should be viewed as a characteristic of the prevailing society, rather than of particular groups or individuals, and interventions should be targeted accordingly.

The mechanisms underlying the diffusion process require further elaboration. Skog's (1985) study of collective drinking behaviour points to the need for investigating the precise ways in which drinkers influence other drinkers and non-drinkers, and more broadly, how substance users affect other users and non-users. Tying this more closely to the communications model of diffusion, as described by Rogers and others, may lead to new ways of looking at the influence of the social environment on substance use.

Investigating the 'discontinuance' phase of diffusion of a substance, or the diffusion of a less harmful or even protective substance, is important for policy development on substance use. One rare example is Warner's (1989) examination of the effect of the US anti-smoking campaign on adult per capita consumption of cigarettes and subsequent mortality. Warner estimates that this 'interference' with the diffusion process postponed almost 800 000 deaths between 1964 and 1985, and an additional two million future deaths to the year 2000. Similar studies of the effect of tax increases on alcohol or of other harm-reduction strategies could provide useful information for policy makers.

Study of the diffusion of non-alcoholic beverages, such as mineral and spring waters, as well as de-alcoholized beverages, and the extent to which they are replacing alcoholic beverages, especially in recent cohorts of drinkers, would provide useful information. The extent to which new beverages replace existing choices or are simply additive is an important question for policymakers.

USING THE DIFFUSION MODEL FOR PREVENTION

Knowledge of patterns of diffusion and discontinuance for substance use in particular groups allows intervention at critical points. Primary prevention may be most important in early stages before the initial steep increase occurs. An example of this approach is the current effort to ban chewing tobacco in some countries before it becomes entrenched. Encouraging quitting and preventing initiation at the beginning of the discontinuance phase may produce much greater payoff than doing so towards the end, when levelling off has already begun. Thus, steep tax measures, as have occurred in Canada during the 1980s, led to a steeper decrease in cigarette smoking than in the USA, which continued with a more liberal taxation policy.

Artificially controlling the distribution of a substance, such as a new psychoactive drug, may be a useful application of this model. Holding back consumption to the early stage of adoption, until sufficient information is available to assess potential problems, could be an important way of preventing widespread problems with a new drug. This can be achieved by placing geographical limitations on prescribing or limiting the number of physicians who can prescribe it.

In the addictions field, there are applications beyond patterns of use in general populations that are potentially useful. These include the diffusion of harm-reduction strategies, such as needle-exchange programmes, among drug addicts; the diffusion of treatment and community-based strategies for preventing alcohol and tobacco-related problems; the diffusion of information about smoking cessation programmes among physicians; and the diffusion of policy approaches to alcohol and tobacco control among public health units and community agencies.

Specific components of the diffusion model can be used in designing specific prevention and intervention efforts. To reduce needle-sharing and introduce needle-exchange programmes, several kinds of information should be gathered. What are the perceived benefits of the current and projected behaviours? What informal communication networks exist in the drug-using community? Is that community centralized or decentralized? What literacy levels characterize users? How complicated is the new method, compared to the old? Can users try it out without commitment? Will users be able to observe other users trying it out? Are there key individuals who function as important role models in the user community?

The introduction of bans on cigarette smoking in public places is a good example, although probably unintentional, of how diffusion can accelerate the discontinuance phase. The observability of smoking is sharply reduced, which functions both to decrease cues for smoking among smokers and to provide non-smoking role models for young people who have not yet taken up smoking. Finding a place to smoke has become more complicated and is often subject to social condemnation. As a smoking friend who cannot smoke at work or at home recently observed, 'There are no more good cigarettes,' meaning the ones at work with a coffee and the ones at home after a meal. Having to stand in the cold to smoke is an aversive experience and not conducive to the spread of smoking. Furthermore, smokers tend to socialize with other smokers, which restricts the opportunity to spread the habit to non-smokers.

In the alcohol field, the introduction of de-alcoholized beer can be analysed in terms of the diffusion model. Concerns have been raised about blurring the distinction between alcoholic and non-alcoholic beverages, especially in the minds of young people. This has been expressed as a fear that easier and less expensive access to non-alcoholic beverages may increase the observability and familiarity of alcoholic beverages and hence provide an easy transition to drinking alcohol at an earlier age.

It is not hard to understand how changes in consumption can be influenced by changes in fashion and changes in simple economic factors. Yet, real world changes are the result of changes at several levels and factors that interact with each other. Developing approaches to slowing increases in use or preventing the introduction of new substances or existing substances to new populations requires consideration of all levels of factors affecting diffusion, and an appreciation of their effect on individual behaviour. A young person contemplating their first drink of alcohol is subject to persuasive factors, including friends, availability, and the perceived status attached to drinking. Aversive factors may be limited to fear of parents finding out. Health concerns are unlikely to be salient at that stage. At later periods of use, higher income may increase the ease of purchase, yet the experience of alcohol-related problems may have a deterrent effect. At all stages of use, the individual is faced with risks and benefits that affect choices about use. Using diffusion theory, those interested in prevention must look at ways of affecting the risk–benefit equation. Education about substance-use problems has little effect unless students increase their perception of increased harm and believe it applies to themselves.

CONCLUSIONS

The widespread application of the diffusion model attests to its utility in adding to our understanding of the adoption of new behaviours, techniques, and products. Its application in the field of substance use is particularly important. Substance use is an area in which aetiology is a major area of investigation and public concern, and results of research on the causes of different trends and patterns of use are often applied quite speedily in programmes, policymaking, and treatment efforts. Using the diffusion model to explain patterns of behaviour has the potential to eliminate many false leads and unproductive approaches. Further, it provides a broad perspective of human behaviour and addictions that encourages new thinking and investigation.

REFERENCES

Ashton, H. and Stepney, R. (1982). *Smoking: psychology and Pharmacology.* London: Tavistock Publications, London.

Barnett, H. G. (1953). *Innovation.* McGraw-Hill, New York.

Bell, D. S. and Champion, R. A. (1976). *Monitoring drug use in New South Wales*, Part 3. Division of Health Service Research, Health Commission of New South Wales, Sydney, Australia.

Blackford, L. St Clair. (1977). *Summary report—surveys of student drug use, San Mateo County, California: alcohol—amphetamines—barbiturates, heroin, LSD, marijuana, tobacco.* Department of Public Health and Welfare, San Mateo County California.

Brown, L. A. (1981). *Innovation diffusion: a new perspective.* Methuen, New York.

Coleman, J. S., Katz, E., and Menzel, H. (1966). *Medical innovation: a diffusion study.* Bobbs—Merrill Company Inc., Indianapolis, USA.

Davis, M. F. (1985). Worksite Health Promotion/Disease Prevention: A Study in the Diffusion of Innovation. Unpublished dissertation, University of Colorado.

Doll, R. and Hill, A. B. (1954). The mortality of doctors in relation to their smoking habits; a preliminary report. *British Medical Journal*, **1**, 1451–5.

Ferrence, R. G. (1989). *Deadly fashion: the rise and fall of cigarette smoking in North America.* Garland Publishing, New York.

Ferrence, R. G. and Kozlowski, L. T. (1990). *Francophone and Anglophone patterns of smoking in Canada: what difference does language make?* Presented to the Annual Meeting of the Canadian Psychological Association, Ottawa, May, 1990.

Godfrey, C. (1989). Factors influencing the consumption of alcohol and tobacco: the use and abuse of economic models. *British Journal of Addiction*, **84**, 1123–38.

Greene, M. H., Kozel, N. J., Hunt, L. G., and Appletree, R. L. (1974). *An assessment of the diffusion of heroin abuse to medium-sized American cities.* Special Action Office Monograph Series A, No. 5, Special Action for Drug Abuse Prevention, Executive Office of the President, Washington DC.

Griliches, Z. (1957). Hybrid corn: an exploration in the economics of techno-logical change, *Econometrica*, **25**, 501–23.

Hughes, P. H. and Crawford, G. A. (1972). A contagious disease model for research and intervening in heroin epidemics. *Archives of General Psychiatry*, **27**, 149–55.

Létourneau, G. (1989). *Francophones and smoking*. Health and Welfare Canada, Ministry of Supply and Services Canada, Cat. No. H39–157/1989E.

Lewit, E. M. and Coate, D. (1982). The potential for using excise taxes to reduce smoking. *Journal of Health Economics*, **1**, 121–45.

Malecki, E. J. (1977). Firms and innovation diffusion: examples from banking, *Environment and Planning*, **9**, 1291–305.

Musto, D. F. (1989). Evolution of American attitudes toward substance abuse. In *Prenatal Abuse of Licit and Illicit Drugs* (ed. H. E. Hutchings), pp. 3–7. Annals of the New York Academy of Sciences, **562**, NY.

Musto, D. F. (1992). America's first cocaine epidemic: what did we learn? pp. 3–15. In *Clinician's guide to cocaine addiction: theory, research and treatment*, (ed. T. R. Kosten and H. D. Kleber), pp. 3–15. The Guilford Substance Abuse Series. Guilford Press, New York.

Pfau, M., Van Bockern, S., and Kang, J. G. (1992). Use of inoculation to promote resistance to smoking initiation among adolescents. *Communication Monographs*, **59**, 213–30.

Pitcher, B. L., Hamblin, R. L., and Miller, J. L. L. (1978). The diffusion of collective violence, *American Sociological Review*, **43**, 23–35.

Robb, J. H. (1986). Smoking as an anticipatory rite of passage: Some socio-logical hypotheses on health-related behaviour. *Social Sciences and Medicine*, **23**, 621–7.

Rogers, E. M. and Shoemaker, F. F. (1971). *Communication of innovations: a cross-cultural approach*, 2nd edn. The Free Press, New York.

Rogers, E. M. (with Shoemaker, F. F.) (1983). *Diffusion of Innovations*, 3rd edn. The Free Press, New York.

Russell, M. A. H. (1971). Cigarette smoking: natural history of a dependence disorder. *British Journal of Medical Psychology*, **44**, 1–16.

Skog, O.-J. (1985): The collectivity of drinking cultures: A theory of the dis-tribution of alcohol consumption. *British Journal of Addiction*, **80**, 83–99.

Sloan, F. A., Valvona, J., Perrin, J. M., and Adamache, K. W. (1986). Dif-fusion of surgical technology: An exploratory study. *Journal of Health Economics*, **5**, 31–61.

Tarde, G. (1903). *The laws of imitation*. H. Holt and Co., New York.

Tornatzky, L. G., Eveland, J. D., Boylan, M. G., Hetzner, W. A., Johnson, E. C., Roitman, D., and Schneider, J. (1983). *The process of technological innova-tion: reviewing the literature*. National Science Foundation, Washington DC.

USHHS (US Department of Health and Human Services) (1980). *The health consequences of smoking for women: a report of the Surgeon General*. Office on Smoking and Health, Rockville, MD, USA..

Warner, K. (1989). Effects of the antismoking campaign: An update. *America Journal of Public Health*, **79**, 144–51.

11

Ideological beliefs influence the feasibilities for policy change

CHARLES R. SCHUSTER *

According to national public opinion polls, drug abuse emerged in the latter part of the 1980s as the number one ethical, moral, legal, social, and public health problem that faced the United States of America. Drug abuse *per se* cannot be divorced from the multiplicity of personal, familial, communal, and national conditions which gave rise to our latest drug abuse 'epidemic' and the often tragic personal, familial, communal, and national consequences which it has spawned. Since different members of our pluralistic society conceptualize this multifaceted problem in different ways, the social and public health policies suggested for its solution are diverse and often contradictory. Further, as is the case with most contentious areas of human behaviour, there is often an inverse relationship between the passion with which people express their views about a policy and the availability of evidence supporting its effectiveness. It is with trepidation that a scientist enters this arena. Ideologies to a considerable extent set the possibilities for policy change.

THOUGHTS ON THE NATURE OF THE PROBLEM

Scientists are rarely policy makers in the Federal Government of the United States of America, except within the narrow confines of the

* The views expressed herein are the views of the author and do not necessarily reflect the official position of the National Institute on Drug Abuse or any other part of the US Department of Health and Human Services. From March 1986 until January 1992 Dr Schuster served as the Director of the National Institute on Drug Abuse which is part of the Public Health Service in the United States Government.

governance of science. Policy makers are, by and large, individuals who are elected to congress or appointed by the President to enact policies emanating from or at least consistent with the platform upon which he or she was elected. Thus, policies are determined by many different factors in addition to scientific data. Political and economic considerations, as well as ethical and moral judgments enter into the decision-making process of policy makers. Which of these influences predominates depends not only upon the issue but as well, the 'Zeitgeist' of the society. The principal role of the scientist is to provide, where possible, scientific data to assist in the policy-making process, recognizing that only rarely will such contributions determine the outcome.

As has been stressed previously (Moore and Gerstein 1981), the most fundamental determinant of policy is the manner in which the problem is conceptualized. Policies generally flow from relatively simplified 'conceptions' which determine the 'governing ideas' from which specific instances of policy are derived. If drug abuse is conceived as the expression of weak moral constraint leading to unfettered hedonism then the 'governing ideas and derivative policies' flow almost inexorably. On the other hand, if biobehavioural sciences can amass sufficient, compelling evidence that drug abuse is most usefully conceptualized as a chronic relapsing disease, similar in its characteristics to morbid obesity or arthritis, the policies adopted to control this problem will be quite different. The conceptualization of drug abuse as a disease similar to arthritis encounters the objection that it appears, at least in the beginning, to be self-inflicted. It is interesting to speculate that an important consequence of the findings that there is a genetic predisposition for the development of at least certain forms of alcoholism (Cloninger *et al.* 1981; Pickens *et al.* 1991) has been to change the conception of this condition being a sign of moral weakness to that of a disease. Further, the finding that there is a genetic basis for a predisposition for alcoholism diminishes the personal responsibility for the development of the problem. There is no doubt that this lies behind the vigorous efforts to demonstrate a similar genetic basis for other forms of drug abuse and dependence.

The complication for the area of drug abuse policy is that, in fact, drug abuse can be conceived as both a problem of morality and a public health problem. Thus, both conceptions of the problem are applicable, but are appropriate at different stages in the natural history of the development of the disease. Moral sanctions can deter individuals from ever experimenting with drugs. High school seniors who have a high degree of involvement with formalized religion, for example, have low prevalence rates for any form of illicit drug use (Bachman *et al.* 1988, 1990). However, only a minority of youth in the USA has a significant involvement with formalized religion. Further, the high prevalence of psychopathology, especially antisocial personality, found in drug abusers, sets limits on the population which are amenable to drug abuse prevention through moral constraints (Regier *et al*. 1990). Finally, where there is a breakdown in the structure and functioning of the family and community, children may not be given the ethical and moral training that would deter drug use. If such ethical and moral constraints are ineffective or absent, for whatever reason, and the individual escalates from drug experimentation to dysfunctional use and dependence, the problem changes. Then it is most usefully conceptualized as a public health problem and the individual as afflicted with the disease of drug dependence. At this stage of drug dependence, moral constraints alone are as likely to be effective as they would be in the treatment of arthritis. Indeed, one goal of treatment for drug abuse could be conceived as engendering a state in which ethical and moral constraints against illicit drug use can be effective in maintaining abstinence.

Unfortunately, even when the advocates for these alternative ways of conceptualizing drug abuse see the policies as applicable to different stages in the development of a drug abuse problem (or to different portions of the population) they see them as antagonistic. In part this is because it is not entirely clear where in the progression of the developing problem of drug abuse the individual becomes insensitive to ethical and moral forces and must be approached with therapeutic interventions. Further, there is a concern, by advocates on both sides, that granting the validity of the other conceptualization will—weaken the support for their position by the general public and by policy makers in particular. Finally, those advocating a moralistic conception of the problem of drug abuse are concerned that the effectiveness of moral constraints against drug use will be diminished if the emphasis becomes one of avoiding the disease of drug dependence or its consequences, as opposed to avoiding all illicit drug use. What has transpired because of this inflexibility is that our present policies are a mixture of those derived from a moralistic conception of drug abuse and others from a public health conception of the problem. This leads to such seemingly contradictory policies as a ban on needle- and syringe-exchange programmes at the same time that bleach is dispensed to intravenous drug users to sterilize their injection paraphernalia.

The attempt to develop a science-base for our public health approaches to controlling drug abuse is complicated by the fact that significant portions of our society conceptualize this problem in moralistic terms. This has repercussions at the most fundamental level, such as the degree to which society is willing to support scientific studies of the nature of drug abuse, its prevention, and treatment. At a hearing held by the House Appropriation Committee in 1990, the Administrator of the Alcohol, Drug Abuse, Mental Health Administration was asked by the Chairman of the Committee—what does science have to do with drug abuse? A great deal if one views it as a public health problem— very little if it is viewed as a problem of morality.

The analysis of alcohol and public policy developed by Moore and Gerstein (1981) is equally applicable to drug abuse policy. They emphasize that if we as scientists are to be maximally effective in influencing policy decisions then we must recognize the fundamental importance of the way the problem is conceptualized. The general public and our elected officials deal with TV sound bites and slogans which are the governing ideas dictated by the way the problem is conceived. If we are to influence policy we must influence the conceptualization, which in turn determines the slogans—everything else will then fall in place.

IDEOLOGIES AS A CONSTRAINT ON RESEARCH METHODS

There are some policy issues which arise because certain scientific practices clash with the ethical or religious beliefs of a segment of society. For example, research using human fetal tissue is considered by many scientists to be an essential part of their activities. This research has generated great controversy because of ethical and moral concerns over the use of fetal tissue obtained by surgical abortions. It is argued that the decision to have an abortion might be made more likely by the knowledge that the aborted fetal tissue could be of value to treat another human suffering from an incurable disease.

The use of animals in research is another issue where the methods used by scientists are generating a controversial public policy issue. In the USA we have seen the development over the past decade of a formidable animal rights movement which has increasingly succeeded in restricting the use of animals for biobehavioral research. The overarching conceptualization of the animal advocacy groups is that all life forms are of equal value and therefore enjoy equal rights. This is best illustrated by the oft-quoted statement by Ingrid Newkirk (Director: People for the Ethical Treatment of Animals): 'Animal liberationists do not separate out the human animal. A rat is a pig is a dog is a boy'. Obviously, if this conceptualization is granted then it becomes difficult to justify a policy that allows the use of any animal species for scientific research even though it may improve the health and quality of life for humans. Fortunately, this view of the equality of all life forms has not found favour among the general public, and the animal advocacy groups have been forced to change their attack on animal research. The use of animals for drug abuse research has been targeted because this area is perceived as more vulnerable than animal research on cancer, heart disease, Alzheimer's, and so on. This vulnerability stems from the fact that many individuals see the problem of drug abuse as a moral issue, and believe that people become drug addicts because of their own moral failings. This conception makes it difficult to justify the use of animals for research to study a condition that is 'self-inflicted'. Why should animals have to suffer to help an individual who wilfully experimented with illicit drugs? Thus once more the conceptualization of drug abuse as a problem of morality has been brought forth, in this instance to make it more difficult to justify the use of animal research to better understand and treat this condition. The latest attempt to destroy drug-abuse animal research is to conceptualize the problem of drug abuse as a social problem which is unique to human society and therefore not amenable to analysis through animal research. Bumper stickers stating that animal research in the area of drug abuse is 'scientific fraud' are the latest in the attempts to decrease public support for animal research. In all of these instances policies concerning the appropriateness of the use of animals in drug abuse research may be seen as derivative from the ways in which the problem of drug abuse is viewed.

In the USA we also conduct drug-abuse research using human volunteers. This practice also poses its own unique ethical and moral questions. If we want to study the human pharmacology of cocaine, dare we administer this drug to humans in controlled laboratory conditions to study its effects? Cocaine is a drug on which our society is expending vast resources to stop people using. Yet, scientists feel that to develop effective treatments for cocaine addiction we need the insights which can only be provided by controlled laboratory studies of the effects of cocaine in humans. If we are going to conduct these kinds of experiments, who should the subjects be? Can we use naive people who have never experienced cocaine before and run the risk of addicting them? (It is of interest to note that cocaine has been imbued with such mythical powers to enslave that it cannot be studied in naive human subjects, but amphetamines and opiates can be). We cannot use individuals who are dependent upon cocaine since they cannot give informed consent because, by definition, if they are addicted, they have lost freedom of choice over their drug-taking behaviour. The decision that has been made by the biomedical field, is that individuals who are naive should not be exposed to cocaine for research purposes nor should we use people who are addicted. However, there are people who use cocaine on an intermittent basis, and who will freely volunteer to come into a laboratory setting to receive controlled doses of cocaine.

The current accepted policy is that these non-addicted 'casual' users of cocaine can serve as subjects in cocaine studies.

There are those who contend that cocaine should not be given to human research subjects under any conditions (Nahas 1990), and so we find ourselves with a problem. The animal advocacy groups do not want scientists to use animals in drug-abuse research and suggest that we use humans. Others feel that it is unethical and unsafe for scientists to use humans in drug-abuse research. -To date, we have preserved the right to do both, but, with increasing restrictions and additional costs engendered by bureaucratic regulations.

QUESTIONS SURROUNDING COMPULSORY TREATMENT

Policy controversies often emanate from the conflict over two passionately held values. For example, the values might be those of individual liberty and privacy versus protection of the individual, as well as his or her family, community or society, from their own destructive use of drugs. There are many instances where these kinds of value-clashes occur in the area of drug abuse. Research often has implications which stimulate such situations.

For many years it has been clear that the dependence-producing properties of opiates can be blocked by an adequate dose of naloxone or its longer-acting analogue naltrexone (Jaffe and Martin 1990). The problem has been that many heroin-dependent patients will not take these medications on a regular basis. A variety of behavioural procedures have been developed to increase compliance for the daily use of naltrexone. This has met with success in a limited portion of the population. Many of these procedures have involved so-called therapeutic contingency contracts in which the patient agrees to take naltrexone and to remain drug-free (as demonstrated by drug-free urine samples), with failure to do so resulting in the loss of their right to practise medicine or some other profession (Crowley 1984). Where patients have 'something to lose' as well as a community which provides positive reinforcement for continued compliance with the therapeutic contract, patients are successful. Unfortunately, such patients constitute the minority of heroin users, with most having little to lose and a community which encourages their taking of heroin rather than abstinence.

Epidemiological research has shown that most heroin users come under the control of the criminal justice system at some point in their lives, either because of arrest for possession of illicit drugs or the crimes they commit to finance their drug purchases (Nurco *et al*. 1985). These occasions can be utilized as opportunities to enrol people into treatment for their drug problem. One approach that is currently being investigated is for heroin addicts who run up against the criminal justice system for non-violent crimes, to be given a suspended jail sentence if they agree to enter treatment and take naltrexone on a regular basis (McLellan 1992). Failure to comply with these conditions would result in their jail sentence immediately being activated. This policy has faced relatively little resistance, in large part, because our jails and prisons are grossly overcrowded and costly to expand. A second proposal, however, has generated a great deal more controversy. This controversy has resulted from the development of a long-acting depot formulation of naltrexone which effectively blocks the effects of opiates for a 4–6 week period. Since patient compliance is less of an issue (that is, they only have to receive the injection every six weeks) it has been suggested that prisoners leaving prison, who have in the past rapidly relapsed to heroin use, be given the naltrexone depot as a condition of their release. It is fairly certain that most people faced with this situation would agree to take the depot naltrexone. However, once the individual is released from prison they may not be quite so agreeable.

The policy question then becomes whether society has the right to force them into compliance. From a practical viewpoint since the naltrexone has to be given only once every 4–6 weeks it is conceivable that a court mandated programme enforcing compliance could be implemented. But is it acceptable to medicate people against their will under these circumstances? Courts in the USA have ruled that if a patient is 'competent' they must make the decision whether or not to take a particular medication on the basis of the full disclosure of the relative risks and expected benefits of that medication. These same considerations apply to people who are confined in prisons and mental hospitals, and even to those involved in compulsory treatment, if they are judged competent to make informed decisions about their treatment. On the other hand, if an individual is judged to be 'mentally incompetent' to make such decisions, they may be medicated without their consent.

It is the current opinion of constitutional lawyers in the USA that although mandatory treatment for drug abuse is constitutional, compulsory medication is not. It could be argued that the heroin-dependent person is not 'mentally competent' to make a free decision regarding their treatment since their dependence limits their choices. Further, it could be argued that the untreated heroin addict represents a danger to themselves and others because of the crimes they commit, as well as their role in the spread of infections such as HIV. Thus, the policy clash unfolds with those who conceptualize the disease of drug dependence as one which limits the 'competence' of the heroin-dependent individual to make a free and informed choice regarding their use of a medication, versus those who fear the encroachment of the state on the individuals right to privacy and protection from cruel and unusual punishment. The policies that ultimately emerge will be heavily influenced, once again, by the way we think of the problem of drug dependence.

MORAL CONSTRAINTS ON HARM MINIMIZATION

It is clear that there are policies based upon non-scientific considerations which can promote or curtail the activities of scientists. For example, the space race of the 1960s was largely based upon a desire of people in the USA to 'keep up with the Russians', not because we were inherently interested in getting into outer space. That kind of attitude, on the part of the public, had an incredible positive impact on the development of physics and many other areas of the physical sciences. Tragically, there are other areas in which there are attitudes and resulting policy decisions which have a negative impact upon science.

One of the most poignant problems we face today are children born with HIV infection. In many such instances the mother is an intravenous drug user or the partner of an intravenous drug user. It is generally agreed that the principal vector of spread of HIV infection into the heterosexual population has been through the heterosexual activity of intravenous drug users. Once a pool of HIV-infected individuals is established in the heterosexual population the infection can rapidly spread if appropriate precautions are not taken. Currently, the spread of HIV infection in the heterosexual population is the most rapidly growing vector in the USA. There are two actions which could be taken to limit the spread of HIV infection; that is to provide an easily accessible source of sterile needles and syringes to intravenous drug users and to adopt an aggressive public education campaign to make condom use as routine as the use of car seat belts. Although these measures have not been proven to limit the spread of HIV infection, it seems obvious that they have a high enough probability of at least limited success to justify their being implemented and evaluated. Neither of these approaches has unanimous support in the USA today. The Public Health Service recently decided to cancel a public education programme on the use of condoms to deter the spread of HIV infection. It is the current position of the Public Health Service that federally supported public education campaigns should stress sexual abstinence in the unmarried, rather than condom use, to avoid the appearance that the government is encouraging premarital sex.

There is also a great concern regarding the appropriateness of the federal government's involvement in needle- and syringe-exchange programmes. Recent epidemiological evidence collected in the USA suggests that the legal availability of sterile needles and syringes among diabetic heroin addicts results in a significantly lower prevalence rate of HIV infection (Nelson *et al.* 1991). These data suggest the efficacy of programmes which would make sterile needles and syringes available to intravenous drug users as a way of limiting the spread of infectious diseases such as AIDS. Nevertheless, in the congressional appropriations for the Public Health Service in 1988 (Public Law 100–607—Nov. 4, 1988) the following was inserted:

None of the funds provided under this Act shall be used to provide individuals with hypodermic needles or syringes so that such individuals may use illegal drugs, unless the Surgeon General of the United States determines that a demonstration needle exchange program would be effective in reducing drug abuse and the risk that the public will become infected with the etiological agent for acquired immune deficiency syndrome.

There are two problems with this statement: first, how can the Surgeon General determine, in advance of a controlled investigation, of the efficacy of a needle-exchange programme that the programme is effective in decreasing the further spread of HIV infection? Second, the bill states that the needle-exchange programme must not only be effective in decreasing the spread of HIV infection, but must also be effective in reducing drug abuse. No one has ever suggested that needle-exchange programmes would decrease drug abuse (although critics of these programmes contend that they will increase drug abuse by making it safer and more acceptable). It is clear that this is thinly disguised language to prevent the establishment of needle-exchange programmes using federal funds.

This position on needle- and syringe-exchange programmes must be understood as being derived from the concept that drug abuse is a moral problem which can best be contained by societies' adoption of the governing idea of 'zero tolerance for illicit drug use'. If we have zero tolerance for drug use then we cannot have federal funds being used to make it safer for individuals to use drugs. The argument that is given is that we would be sending a 'double message' to the children in our society if we tell them that drug use is unacceptable, but we provide the equipment to make it safer for drug addicts to use illicit drugs. Although the current Appropriations Bill for the Public Health Service no longer contains the language prohibiting the funding of needle- and syringe-exchange programmes, it is still the policy that federal funds cannot be used to support needle-exchange programmes.

THE PREGNANT WOMAN

A second problem in the area of drug abuse that tugs on the heart strings of America is that of the pregnant addict and the problems which her continued drug use pose to the fetus and to her ability to provide a nurturing environment postnatally. In the USA we are constantly regaled in the press with horrifying stories of thousands of unadoptable 'crack babies' being abandoned by their drug-crazed adolescent mothers, and doomed to a childhood of uncaring foster homes and schools which their drug-induced intellectual impairment makes a source of constant frustration. Estimates of the prevalence of this problem vary widely (13 750 to 375 000 for the year 1987: Dicker and Leighton, 1991), but it is generally perceived as 'large'. Further, it is not clear what damage to the fetus and neonate are attributable to the mother's use of cocaine as opposed to their concomitant use of tobacco and/or alcohol, poor nutrition, sexually transmitted diseases, and lack of prenatal medical care (Kilbey and Asghar, 1991). In recent years society's frustration with this problem has led to the enactment of state laws which have made the use of drugs during pregnancy an act of child abuse for which the mother may lose custody of the child and/or may face criminal sanctions. In one of the most egregious cases, a physician allowed the fetus to be delivered and immediately took blood samples from the placenta which were sent for analysis for the presence of cocaine. Since the blood coming from the mother through the placenta to the neonate was found to contain cocaine the mother was arrested for the delivery of drugs to a minor (Curriden 1990).

It is of interest to note that the increase in obstetric knowledge and the development of techniques for diagnosing and treating the growing fetus directly, including even surgical procedures, has changed the relationship of the obstetrician to the fetus. In the past, the obstetrician ensured the health of the developing fetus by treating the woman. They essentially constituted one patient. Today, we have a situation in which the woman and the fetus may be viewed as separate patients. Circumstances can, however, develop whereby the mother, as a competent adult, may choose to refuse certain types of medical interventions, or to engage in behaviours which may be detrimental to the health and viability of the fetus, thus placing the physician in an ethical conflict about his or her responsibilities to the 'two patients'. The legal and practical problems faced by the physician with this dilemma are well stated by Nelson and Milliken (1988). They conclude that:

if society and the medical profession are truly interested in enhancing fetal health, their efforts should be directed toward increasing the availability and quality of voluntary prenatal care for all pregnant women and the availability of drug and alcohol rehabilitation programmes and other social services for those pregnant women who need them and discouraging physicians from running to the courthouse for an order forcing a woman to accept treatment she does not want.

Pragmatically, the forced treatment or criminalization of pregnant women who are using illicit drugs will only result in their failing to seek prenatal care, a condition which is far worse for their developing fetus. Clinical research (Wapner and Finnegan 1981) has shown that placental infections are common among drug-using pregnant woman and may be of greater consequence for fetal development than continued drug use. Thus, any policy that makes it less likely that drug-using pregnant women will seek prenatal care is clearly counterproductive, from a public health perspective.

WHAT PRICE RATIONALITY?

Although science may not be determinative of policy it could, and should, be used to a much greater extent to evaluate the impact of drug-abuse policy. Where policy changes involve decisions about the allocation of major resources it is incumbent that funding be made available to evaluate whether the policy is producing the desired outcome in a cost-effective manner. The steps for doing this are easy, at least in theory. Where the policy is designed to produce some behavioural change on the part of a target population, we must first define the behaviour or the practice we are trying to change; second, before any policy change takes place we must measure the baseline frequency of the behaviour or practice we are trying to affect; third, we must work with policy makers to ensure that when the policy is implemented that an appropriate process evaluation be conducted to determine the cost and success of the implementation of the policy; next, after a suitable length of time following the implementation of the policy, changes in the target behaviour should be measured; and finally, the outcome data, the process evaluation and reports of any unpredicted 'side-effects' must be evaluated to determine the extent to which the policy is producing the desired changes in behaviour in a cost-effective manner. Such an evaluation can assist policy makers and the general public in determining whether to maintain the policy, or if further policy change is necessary.

One of the most clear-cut and effective uses of science for policy evaluation is in the case of the changes in the drinking age laws which took place in several states in the USA in the early 1970s. Following the lowering of the minimal age at which alcoholic beverages could be purchased, highway safety statistics showed a significant increase in alcohol-related traffic fatalities in youth. When that policy was reversed, and the legal age for the purchase of alcoholic beverages was raised to 21 the number of traffic fatalities in the age range 16 to 24 went down again (Saffer and Grossman 1987). From a scientific viewpoint, it was a model ABA design experiment. The evidence from these studies was subsequently used in a Supreme Court case to successfully defend the Federal Uniform Drinking Age Act, which called for all states to raise the minimum age at which alcoholic beverages could be purchased to 21. As pointed out by Gordis (1991), science alone did not win the Supreme Court case, rather it was the combination of scientific evidence showing the wisdom of raising the drinking age to 21, along with very impassioned advocacy by the National Council on Alcoholism, 'Remove Intoxicated Drivers', and other advocacy groups which filed *amici curiae* briefs.

There are many other areas in drug-abuse policy where science could be used to assist policy makers in evaluating their success. The effectiveness of pre-employment drug testing as a predictor of which employees would show significantly higher absenteeism, job-turnover rate, health-care costs, and accident rates has been investigated in a prospective study (Normand *et al*. 1990). This study clearly showed that employees who tested positive for marihuana in a pre-employment urine drug test had higher rates of absenteeism and job turnover rates then employees hired at the same time who tested negative. It should be noted that in this case the investigators did not imply that marijuana was a cause of the increased absenteeism or job turnover rates, rather that the positive urine screen for marijuana was simply used as a predictor. An analysis of the costs of the urine drug testing procedures and the savings affected by screening-out potential employees who used marijuana showed that such screening would save employers a significant amount of money. Although a policy of screening-out potential employees who test positive for marijuana makes sense from a corporate viewpoint, it remains to be determined whether it has a positive impact on society. The ideas of 'user responsibility' and 'zero tolerance for drug use' which govern current federal drug policy favour such practices. It is the belief of the current federal drug-abuse policy makers that drug testing in the workplace will not only decrease costly consequences but will also act as a powerful disincentive for the use of illicit drugs. Unfortunately, there is currently no way of evaluating this contention nor any plans to conduct a controlled study to determine the extent to which this policy is having the desired outcome. There are many other areas of drug-abuse policy where small-scale investigations of the impact of policy change could be accomplished before widespread implementation of the policy. Using this strategy, science, could, at minimal cost, add immensely to the effectiveness of our legislative and regulatory policy making.

Society has made a substantial investment in the development of a science base for understanding the aetiology of drug abuse, its consequences, and its prevention and treatment. Our knowledge base has increased substantially over the past decade in all of these areas. It is incumbent upon scientists to make elected officials, other public policy makers, and the general public aware that this science base can be utilized to conceptualize more usefully the multifaceted problems associated with drug abuse, frame policy change in a manner that can be evaluated, and assist in the assessment of the success of drug-abuse policy.

REFERENCES

Bachman, G., Johnston, L., O'Malley, P., and Humphrey, R. (1988). Explaining the recent decline in marijuana use: Differentiating the effects of perceived risks, disapproval and life style factors. *Journal of Health and Social Behavior*, **29**, 92–102.

Bachman, G., Johnston, I., and O'Malley, P. (1990). Explaining the recent decline in cocaine use: Differentiating the effects of perceived risk, disapproval and lifestyle factors. *Journal of Health and Social Behavior*, **31**, 173–84.

Cloninger, C. R., Bohman, M., and Sigvardsson, S. (1981). Inheritance of alcohol abuse: Cross-fostering analysis of adopted men. *Archives of General Psychiatry*, **38**, 861–8.

Crowley, T. J. (1984). Contingency contracting treatment of drug-abusing physicians, nurses, and dentists. *National Institute on Drug Abuse Research Monograph Series*, **46**, 68–83.

Curriden, M. (1990). Holding mom accountable. *American Bar Association Journal*, **50**, 4.

Dicker, M. and Leighton, E. A. (1991). Trends in diagnosed drug problems among newborns: United States, 1979–1987. *Drug and Alcohol Dependence*, **28**, 151–65.

Gordis, E. (1991). From science to social policy: an uncertain road. *Journal of Studies of Alcohol*, **52**, 101–9.

Jaffe, J. H. and Martin, W. R.. (1990). Opioid analgesics and antagonists. In *Goodman and Gilman: The pharmacological basis of therapeutics*, 8th edn. (ed. A. G. Gilman, T. W. Rall, A. S. Nies, and P. Taylor), pp. 485–521. Pergamon Press, New York.

Kilbey, M. M. and Asghar, K. (ed.) (1991). *Methodological issues in controlled studies on effects of prenatal exposure to drug abuse*. National Institute on Drug Abuse Research Monograph Series, No. 114.

McLellan, A. T. (1992). How effective is drug abuse treatment: Compared to what? In *Addictive states* (ed. J. Jaffe and C. O'Brien), pp. 231–52. Raven Press, New York.

Moore, M. H. and Gerstein, D. R. (ed.) (1981). *Alcohol and public policy: beyond the shadow of prohibition*. National Academy Press, Washington, DC.

Nahas, G. G. (1990). The experimental use of cocaine in human subjects. *Bulletin on Narcotics*, **42**, 57–62.

Nelson, K. E., Vlahov, D., Cohn, S., Lindsay, A., Solomon, L., and Anthony, J. C. (1991). Human immunodeficiency virus infection in diabetic intravenous drug users. *Journal of the American Medical Association*, **266**, 2259–61.

Nelson, L. J. and Milliken, N. (1988). Compelled medical treatment of pregnant women. *Journal of the American Medical Association*, **259**, 1060–6.

Normand, J., Salyards, S. D., and Mahoney, J. J. (1990). An evaluation of preemployment drug testing. *Journal of Applied Psychology*, **75**, 629–39.

Nurco, D. N., Ball, J. C., Shaffer, J. W., and Hanlon, T. E. (1985). The criminality of narcotic addicts. *Journal of Nervous and Mental Disease*, **73**, 94–102.

Pickens, R. W., Svikis, D. S., McGue, M., Lykken, D. T., Heston, L. L., and Clayton, P. J. (1991). Heterogeneity in the inheritance of alcoholism: A study of male and female twins. *Archives of General Psychiatry*, **48**, 19–28.

Regier, D. A., Farmer, M. E., Rae, D. S., Locke, B. Z., Keith, S. J., Judd, L. L., and Goodwin, F. K. (1990). Comorbidity of mental disorders with alcohol and other drug abuse. *Journal of the American Medical Association*, **264**, 2511–18.

Saffer, H. and Grossman, M. (1987). Beer taxes, the legal drinking age, and youth motor vehicle fatalities. *Journal of Legal Studies*, **16**, 351–74.

Wapner, R. J. and Finnegan, L. P. (1981). Perinatal aspects of psychotropic drug abuse. In *Perinatal medicine* (ed R. J. Bolognese, R. H. Schwartz, and J. Schneider), pp. 383–417. Williams and Wilkins, Baltimore, MD.

Part IV.

Processes of change: making the connection between theory and clinical practice

12

Multiple indicators of change: can we identify the dimensions?

JOHN STRANG

Change is central to our consideration of interventions with addictive behaviour—but what change? Whether our interest is in addiction as a 'progressive disease' (see Chapter 6) or in adaptation of the neuro-receptor (see Chapter 3), this is necessarily accompanied by a sense of progression from point A to point B. But are we sure we know the grid reference points for A and B so as to be able either to chart progress or to influence the extent of progress? Likewise, if we are considering some treatment (or other intervention), then we will need an awareness of the location of points A and B if we are to be able to gauge the extent to which recovery has occurred, or progression has been arrested—accompanied by a fuller understanding of the changes we would expect to have occurred in the untreated condition.

Where are points A and B, and the factors which influence pro-gression or non-progression between the two? And what are the dif-ferent points A and B which may exist? In examining this issue, our consideration will need to encompass those changes which we regard as disease progression or deterioration, as well as those which are regarded as recovery or improvement (whether by self-help, maturing out, or by treatment). Whether they are regarded as good or bad changes is a separate issue, on which the judgement may change over time, whereas the robustness of our observations on the change which has occurred should be capable of standing the test of time—as Bertrand Russell

---

*Some of the material presented in the later part of this chapter is drawn from a discussion document and address prepared by the author for the *Third international conference on the reduction of drug-related harm* (Melbourne, March 1992)

said 'Change is scientific, progress is ethical; change is indubitable, whereas progress is a matter of controversy'.

In some respects, the 'process of change' has become the new organizing idea for the addictions field in recent years. It carries with it the understanding that change is not a single event but a process: this invites consideration of the natural order of this process, and consideration of the points of possible influence (or at least points at which an intervention is more likely to bring about change). Consideration of personal or public health interventions are not, in themselves, then considered as the totality of the intervention, but rather they are considered according to the re-positioning which results from the intervention. If we consider Winick's idea from the early 1960s of 'maturing out' (Winick 1962), then we first need a fuller understanding of this process of 'maturing out', the types of 'maturing out' which we may expect to see, and some indications of the ways in which we may bring about a speeding-up of this natural process (or at least avoid inadvertently slowing it down).

In this chapter, consideration is given to the nature of the change which is the subject of the process. In the first section, the significance of change is explored, some of which changes will be considered as progress. The impact of HIV is then considered, accompanied by examples of how recent policy documents have taken this on board. The next section then looks at treatments covered by the rubric 'harm reduction', and explores the relationship between individual and public health benefit. Finally, consideration is given to the different dimensions of harm which can be identified, and the ways in which these might be measured in future monitoring of change seen in drug takers, or in studies of treatment populations.

WHAT SIGNIFICANCE SHOULD BE ATTACHED TO THE CHANGES OBSERVED?

Negative as well as positive changes

Change does not necessarily mean change for the good. In the policy and treatment arena, it may be as well for us to remember the medical aphorism that the only treatments without side effects are the treatments without good effects either. If we are considering interventions which may confer benefit (the 'wanted effect' described by Lader, this book) then this should be accompanied by a consideration of the harms: that is, consideration of the negative as well as the positive possible changes.

And so we come to the notion that there may be benefits in one area whilst harms occur in another—that there may be a positive change along one dimension whilst there is negative change along another. The long-term prescribing of benzodiazepines perhaps illustrates this point— there is evidently a perceived short-term benefit (and possibly medium-term and even long-term benefit), not only by virtue of their pharmacological anxiolytic properties, but also when the Valium acts like oil on troubled waters—the storm may still rage or the hidden reef may still loom, but there is, at least for now, a temporary calm. There are benefits, and there are harms or costs. So what has changed to bring about the reduced acceptability of long-term prescribing of benzodiazepines? Certainly our level of understanding of the existence of harms may have improved, but we have also seen a re-calculation by society as a whole of the cost-benefit analysis. Even if there had been a constant level of scientific knowledge, we would probably have seen, in recent years, a reassessment by society of the importance it attaches to the various dimensions of benefit and harm which are associated with the benzodiazepines. Consider also the long-term prescribing of oral methadone in methadone maintenance programmes: from the single perspective of addiction or dependence, the ongoing provision of daily supervised supplies of oral methadone over periods of years must surely be an institutionalization and perpetuation of the opiate dependence itself, but there is now impressive evidence, over several decades, of benefits which may be accrued in dimensions other than dependence, such as the stability of family life, employment, criminality, and so on (for a recent review, see Ball and Ross 1991). Indeed, Preble and Miller (1977) talk of the heroin addict entering the methadone 'interworld'; at different times, and in different places, this move into the interworld will be considered as a step forward or a step backward.

Perhaps as scientists our task is to chart the various changes, and to assist while society considers whether one or another constellation of changes represents the greater or the lesser progress.

Studying the finer features of change

There is something attractively simple about the move from non-use to use, or the later move to abstinence, as measures of change. However, the reliance on this gross change may result in a failure to consider changes *within* continued use which are nevertheless interesting and important. Does the continued drug use mean continued injecting or not? For example, in the three-year follow-up of drug addicts turned away from treatment, Strang *et al.* (1987) found evidence of considerable diversity in the nature of the continued drug use in the 55 subjects who were still using drugs at follow-up. Virtually all subjects had previously been injecting their drugs, yet by follow-up 20 per cent were no longer injecting, and 22 per cent were injecting only occasionally, despite being part of the cohort who continued to use drugs. Only 4 per cent reported an increase in frequency of injecting. Whilst still on the 'slippery slope', there would appear to be scope for considerable movement up as well as down the slope for at least some individuals.

Similarly, in the current study at the Maudsley (London) into transitions in heroin use, there is extensive evidence in our interviews with more than 400 local heroin users of lasting changes ('transitions') in their route of heroin use: in a preliminary analysis of the first 200 subjects, 89 subjects identified a total of 113 separate transitions, with a ratio of approximately 2:1 between 'onward transitions' (taken to refer to transitions which were deemed to increase the seriousness, such as from smoking to injecting), and 'reverse transitions' (usually from injecting to smoking) (Strang *et al.* 1992). From a separate sample (a treatment sample of 75 subjects on an in-patient unit), Griffiths *et al.* (1992) reported that 45 per cent of subjects reported previous transition from chasing to injecting, whilst 23 per cent reported earlier change from injecting to either chasing or snorting.

A range of changes have previously been measured. For example in the Hartnoll and Mitcheson study comparing intravenous heroin maintenance and oral methadone maintenance, the authors reported on the extent of various different types of change including daily illicit opiate use, daily total opiate use, frequency of injecting, proportion of time with other drug users, crime as a source of income, and number of arrests (Hartnoll *et al.* 1980).

Similarly, the extensive TOPS study in the USA (Treatment Outcome Prospective Study) considered a number of possible changes as measures of treatment outcome—extent of drug and alcohol use, mental health, illegal activities, and employment (or other economic or socially approved productive behaviour) are considered as valid measures in addition to retention in, and completion of, treatment (see Hubbard *et al.* 1984, 1989).

Having made the observations, we are though still unable to conduct a cost–benefit analysis until we know the importance of each positive or negative change. How are weightings to be assigned to reductions in the amount of property crime or crimes of violence against the person (impacts on others), compared with reductions in the damage to home life or physical well-being of the drug user themselves?

THE IMPACT OF HIV

AIDS is forcing a re-evaluation of research, policy, and practice in the drugs field. Perhaps the dimensions of change may remain the same, but the importance which is attached to them by us or by society as a whole may be fundamentally altered by awareness of the risk of HIV infection—not only amongst drug users but also through them to the broader population. As on previous occasions, there may be a tussle between considerations of the public health and considerations of the individual well-being of the drug user.

What are the changes we wish to promote? AIDS has certainly brought about a greater appreciation of benefits other than dose reduction and abstinence (benefits such as the move away from injecting, or at least away from sharing needles and syringes); but it has also brought about a re-allocation of weightings to be attached to personal and public benefits. Consider the statement from the Advisory Council on the Misuse of Drugs (ACMD 1988) in their AIDS and Drug Misuse report, that:

the spread of HIV is a greater danger to individual and public health than drug misuse. Accordingly, we believe that services which aim to minimize HIV risk behaviour by all available means should take precedence in development plans.

This represents not only a re-ordering of our hierarchy of concerns at the level of the individual and his or her behaviour, but also re-establishes the dominant position of public well-being—at least alongside, and possibly above, considerations of individual well-being.

Our task as scientists must surely be to chart the changes, which we may regard as absolute, whilst the task of determining whether these are progress or not (and if so how one progress matches up to another) is a different area of consideration for society as a whole to which we may wish to contribute but where the conclusions will rightly vary as the circumstances themselves vary.

The repositioning of causes for concern which formed the basis of that ACMD report requires careful examination. Policy makers and practitioners (and hence by implication trainers and researchers) were encouraged to consider a hierarchy of causes for concern, and hence a hierarchy of goals for their interventions. The concept of 'intermediate goals' appears in the report, referring to 'goals which fall short of abstinence'. Thus 'we must be prepared to work with those who continue to misuse drugs to help them reduce the risks involved in doing so, above all the risk of acquiring or spreading HIV'. So it was recommended that there should be a re-ordering of society's hierarchy of causes for concern. A great good may be best, but a bit of good may be good enough, especially if the lesser good may be effective more widely, and may be sufficient to bring about benefit in certain key dimensions—in this example, the prevention of acquisition of HIV, and certainly the prevention of its onward transmission. Thus prescribing is seen as potentially:

a useful tool in helping to change the behaviour of some drug misusers either towards abstinence or towards intermediate goals such as a reduction in injecting or sharing. Thus the individual drug user may move, step by step, through the following intermediate goals—(a) the cessation of sharing of equipment; (b) the move from injectable to oral-only drug use; (c) decrease in drug use; and (d) abstinence (ACMD, 1989).

A CASCADE OF PROCESSES OF CHANGE

The provision of treatment to a drug user is thus no longer seen as an intervention which seeks to encourage movement through a single process of change, but might more usefully be considered as seeking to promote movement through a cascade of processes of change (Strang 1990), with each of the intermediate goals representing an end stage within one of the subsidiary processes of change.

In Fig. 12.1, perhaps the cessation of sharing may be the maintenance stage of process No. 1, with the cessation of any injectable use being the maintenance stage of process No. 2, and the cessation of non-prescribed other drug use as the maintenance stage of process No. 3, for example. In their second report on AIDS and Drug Misuse, the ACMD

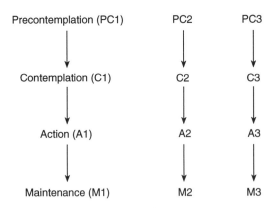

FIG. 12.1 Cascade of processes of change.

considered the possible goals of treatment involving the prescribing of drugs, and emphasized the importance of both working towards an identified goal and measuring the extent of progress towards that goal. Thus they listed the following range of goals which might be considered:

(a) to attract seropositive drug misusers into regular contact with services;

(b) to promote behaviour change away from practices which carry a risk of transmitting HIV infection;

(c) to promote behaviour change in such a way as to maximise personal health and stability;

(d) to encourage compliance with medical treatment including regular check ups and the regular self-administration of zidovudine (AZT).
(ACMD 1989)

Note that the first of these goals is not considered as a sufficient goal in itself, but should rather be considered as the platform on which the others may be founded.

THE RECENT GROWTH OF 'HARM REDUCTION'

The simple measure of abstinence is either considered too imprecise as a measure of change, or may even be considered to be a measure along a different dimension. What then are to be considered the dimensions along which benefit or harm may occur, and according to which we may seek to gauge the extent of change? The recent reviews prompted by AIDS have been accompanied by a great interest in harm-reduction approaches which may be considered at the level of policy or practice (Buning 1990; Stimson 1990; Strang and Farrell 1992). As yet, research has been slow to pick up on this development; there is likely to be greater research activity in the coming years into the various possible reductions in harm, perhaps along the lines of the package of measures of harm which have been put together by Darke, Heather and their colleagues in Sydney in the HIV risk-taking behaviour scale (HRBS) (see, for example, Darke *et al*. 1991). In these instances, the measurement of present behaviour and recent change (and hence the opportunity to measure extent of change over time) concerns the extent of sharing of needles and syringes, and sexual behaviours, and is hence only concerned with the extent of drug use insofar as it is a necessary accompaniment of the risk behaviour or insofar as it may have an influence on the severity or frequency of the risk behaviour.

What changes might constitute harm reduction?

One of the difficulties about measuring changes in harm accrued is that they may not be easily or directly measurable. There may be a convoluted or distorting relationship between the original behaviour and the manifest harm: they may appear at a distance in time (for example the presentation with chronic hepatitis or AIDS several years after the original infection with hepatitis B or HIV), or they may be deliberately concealed (for example as a result of the stigma associated with sexually transmitted diseases), or they may be difficult to identify by virtue of their concentration in hidden populations (for example among prostitutes or among groups who do not have regular access to health care).

What is risk, and how does it relate to harm? Risk relates to the possibility that an event might occur: harm might be seen as the event itself. Harm is presumably our target, and our interest in an existing or proposed strategy should be determined by the extent to which it reduces or increases the amount of harm accrued—considered at either the level of the individual, the community, or society. Sometimes it will be easier to examine changes in risk behaviour, but this will need to be accompanied by a consideration of the reliability of the relationship between the risk and the harm. In these circumstances, risk will sometimes be an acceptable surrogate for the harm already being incurred, or likely to be incurred. Risk and harm may be accrued in different ways. The risk of contracting hepatitis B or HIV from a single episode of sharing needle and syringe can be calculated, but what are the laws which govern how to calculate the cumulative risk as this behaviour continues? Risk per event of drug use is not constant. Indeed, the first occasion of a new type of drug use is probably associated with higher levels of risk for some categories of harm (such as accidental overdose or hepatitis B or HIV infection). Subsequent repeating of the risk behaviour may result in some accumulation of the total risk for the individual, although the additional risk per additional event is likely to be less than that accrued on the first occasion. Thus we are confronted with the paradox that whilst the cumulative total of risk increases with repeated episodes, it may be the case that risk per episode may decrease as the user moves from novice to more informed user. However, it may be that risk per event may later increase again for some individuals as their level of concern, cognitive vigilance, and/or caution may be reduced—for example during periods of greater intoxication, or in association with compromise in atypical circumstances, such as during withdrawals in police custody or prison when the offer of a shared needle and syringe may be uncharacteristically attractive. For such an individual, risk per event will have followed something approximating to a U-shaped curve over time.

Some harms can also be regarded as a single event of harm—for example the risk of a road traffic accident for the drink driver, or the risk of hepatitis B or HIV infection for the injector. Thus a harm-reducing change might be a binary phenomenon—you either have the harm, or you do not. However, other harms are clearly cumulative—for example the liver damage seen with alcoholic cirrhosis. And indeed, although infection with hepatitis B or HIV have been put forward as examples of a single event, actual disease progression may be determined by the cumulative effect of specific co-infections, or by the extent of general immunological insult which then influence the likelihood of progression.

CHANGES IN PERSONAL OR PUBLIC HEALTH

The sought-after changes in personal health are not necessarily the same (and, more frequently, may not have the same priority) as the sought-after changes dictated by a public health perspective. Indeed it is interesting to consider this issue even within the population of drug users—there may be strategies for heroin, alcohol, or benzodiazepine use which confer benefit to the overall population of users whilst disadvantaging a minority within that population. At different times and in different places, the well-being of individual drug users comes to be regarded as less important than the well-being of the broader population of drug users, or of the general population as a whole. Different levels of health strategy need to be considered separately: despite this, the ACMD AIDS and Drug Misuse Report concluded that the necessary changes were required both by personal and public health considerations. And indeed it has been a fortunate and convenient coincidence that many of the proposals for responses to the problems of HIV infection amongst injecting drug users have simultaneously satisfied personal health as well as public health considerations. However, it will not always be so. During the intravenous barbiturate problem in the UK during the 1970s, it is quite possible that the individual well-being of a particular barbiturate injector sitting in the doctor's surgery may have been improved (at least temporarily) by the supervised pre-scribing of some substitute barbiturate; but the perceived longer-term risks and the risk to the broader population of barbiturate injectors appear to have been seen as sufficient to warrant a consensus banning the out-patient prescribing of barbiturates to such drug users. For the injector who accepted these limitations and agreed to in-patient care, it is probable that the forced change of circumstances was associated with beneficial health changes, whereas for the injector who would not accept the limitations, their individual well-being may have deteriorated. We are currently in the middle of a similar dilemma with the intravenous abuse of the benzodiazepines. During the 1980s, temazepam, in the soft liquid-filled capsule form (known to drug users as soft eggs), was extensively injected—using a wide-bore needle due to the substantial viscosity—(for recent commentary, see Strang *et al.* 1993). In response to concerns about this unfolding epidemic and the reports of the associated physical complications, the manufacturers reformulated the preparation in 1989 so that the contents were no longer liquid but were changed to a wax-like gelthix formulation. However, the injecting of the temazepam capsules has continued, with reports of drug users warming the capsule in a microwave, for example, so that the temazepam can be injected through a wide-bore needle. There now appears to be increased morbidity associated with those individuals who inject the drug in this way; but, data are absent on the extent to which this injecting of temazepam has continued. In attempting to measure the extent of change in drug-taking behaviour for the population as a whole, it is necessary not only to look at the evidence of possible increased harm for the individual drug user who continues to inject, but also to look at the extent of total harm accrued by the population. The reformulation may possibly have resulted in increased harm for those individuals who continue to inject temazepam, but a decreased harm for the majority of drug users who may have been deflected on to more established drugs of intravenous use. As yet it is not clear whether the overall change in harm to the population (that is not just the specific ongoing temazepam injectors) has increased or decreased as a result of this control-orientated intervention.

THE DIMENSIONS OF HARM

So what are the dimensions of harm which we may wish to measure as indicators of the extent of change?

At the simplest level, if harm can be accrued as a one-off event or, in other circumstances, may be cumulative, then perhaps this provides us with a single crude dimension of severity of harm. Some harms will be spread across the continuum—for example, the degree of liver damage, the degree of family breakdown, the degree of social dislocation, the degree of criminalization of local community, the degree of economic impact at the national level. (By describing harm along such a continuum, it does not necessarily follow that the affected population will be evenly distributed along this continuum, for it may well be that there will be a clustering of individuals or populations at one or other point on the continuum.) On the other hand, there are some harms (such as infection with HIV or hepatitis B virus) for which the population under study would be found at one or other end of the continuum —and indeed the concept of a continuum becomes meaningless in such a case where there are only two possible positions, which then become categories. However, even with these examples of HIV and hepatitis B infection, it becomes more meaningful to return to the concept of a continuum when we consider the spectrum of disease associated with such infection, with a substantial proportion of the population being under one end of the continuum as asymptomatic seropositives, and with the remaining seropositive population spread along the continuum according to the extent of progression of their disease.

However, this simple explanation presumes that harm is unidimensional, and hence any measurement of change can only be considered according to the extent to which it brings about change in this single dimension. In both the alcohol and drug field the last couple of decades have seen the emergence of the 'problem drinker' and 'problem drug taker', in which the definition includes some attempt to identify the nature of possible harms—in the case of the ACMD definition of the problem drug taker, the 'physical, psychological, social or legal harms'. Following an apparently similar line of thinking, Dorn has recently suggested that four dimensions can reasonably be considered—personal harm, social harm, legal harm, and financial harm (Dorn 1992). As an alternative approach, Newcombe (1992) has recently described a matrix approach to the charting of harm, with the type of harm along one axis (as either health, social, or economic harm) and the level at which the harm is experienced along the other axis (as either individual, community or societal harm). Thus, even by the use of this simple 3 × 3 matrix, our discussion becomes more meaningfully descriptive. If we then move on from this 2-dimensional consideration to consider dimensions for the timing of onset of the harm (short-term through to long-term onset of the harm itself); the duration of the harm (a temporary harm through to a permanent harm); and a measure of the intensity of the harm—then our powers of description become greater, and we have also made significant progress in charting the territory ready for quantification of the harm under consideration.

SHORT-TERM MEASURES OF CHANGE

There is a great temptation to go for measures of profound change (such as abstinence) and to pay much less attention to the measurement of smaller amounts of change, even though the latter measurements may actually be more useful in day-to-day clinical practice (and the research commentary on this practice). For the chest physician, the more absolute change would be the full recovery of his patient with pneumonia, but on an hour-to-hour or day-to-day basis, the more useful measures of change may be the pulse rate and temperature. As an instrument, the thermometer (and the reading of a pulse) give some limited information when giving an isolated reading, but are of much greater value when they are used for the serial measurement of a condition over time: as such, they give an excellent handle on the changes which the physician is observing and wishes to influence. For such reasons, a case can be made in defence of quick and ready measures of some characteristic, such as the Opiate Withdrawal Scale (OWS) (Bradley *et al.* 1987; Gossop 1990) as a measure of the severity of the withdrawal syndrome, or the Drug-Injecting Risk Questionnaire (DIRQ) as a measure of the extent of risk to injectable transmission of HIV or hepatitis B during the last week or month (Strang and Gossop, in preparation).

CONCLUSIONS—THE BALANCE SHEET APPROACH

In conclusion, it may be necessary to see the description of harm or benefit as being multidimensional—of seeing the description of change as requiring multiple indices. Perhaps the only way will be to take a 'balance sheet' perspective in which the harms and benefits (or, less judgmentally, the observed changes) are considered along these different dimensions.

But who has the authority and responsibility for conducting this 'balance sheet' exercise? The scientist can surely contribute to the debate by providing a more thorough report of the changes which are observed in both the natural history and the treated condition, and may provide background information to the context of the consideration. But perhaps, at the end of the day, whilst the description of change will continue to be indubitable and hence a proper area of work for scientists, the identification of benefit or progress is, has been, and always will be a matter of controversy.

REFERENCES

Advisory Council on the Misuse of Drugs (1988). *AIDS and Drugs Misuse Report, Part I*. Her Majesty's Stationery Office, London.
Advisory Council on the Misuse of Drugs (1989). *AIDS and Drugs Misuse Report, Part II*. Her Majesty's Stationery Office, London.

Ball, J. C. and Ross, A. (1991). *The effectiveness of methadone maintenance treatment*. Springer-Verlag, New York.

Bradley, B., Gossop, M., Phillips, G., and Legarda, J. (1987). The development of an opiate withdrawal scale (OWS). *British Journal of Addiction*, **82**, 1139–42.

Buning, E. (1990). The role of harm-reduction programmes in curbing the spread of HIV by drug injectors. In *AIDS and drug misuse: the challenge for policy and practice in the 1990s*, (ed. J. Strang and G. Stimson), pp. 153–61. Routledge, London.

Darke, S., Hall, W., Heather, N., Ward, J., and Wodak, A. (1991). The reliability and validity of a scale to measure HIV risk-taking among intravenous drug users. *AIDS*, **5**, 147–52.

Dorn, N. (1992). Clarifying policy options on drug trafficking. Harm minimisation as distinct from legalisation. In *The reduction of drug related harm* (ed. P. O'Hare, R. Newcombe, A. Matthews, E. Buning, E. Drucker), pp. 108–21. Routledge, London.

Gossop, M. (1990). The development of a short opiate withdrawal scale (SOWS). *Addictive Behaviors*, **15**, 487–90.

Griffiths, P., Gossop, M., Powis, B., and Strang, J. (1992) Extent and nature of transitions of route among heroin addicts in treatment—preliminary data. *British Journal of Addiction*, **87**, 485–92.

Hartnoll, R. L., Mitcheson, M. C., Battersby, A., Brown, G., Ellis, M., Fleming, P., and Hedley, N. (1980). Evaluation of heroin maintenance in controlled trial. *Archives of General Psychiatry*, **37**, 877–84.

Hubbard, R. L., Rachal, J. V., Craddock, S. G., and Cavanaugh, E. R. (1984). Treatment outcome prospective study (TOPS): client characteristics and behaviors before, during and after treatment. In *NIDA research monograph series 51: RAUS Drug abuse treatment evaluation: strategies, progress and prospects* (ed. F. M. Tims and J. P. Ludford), pp. 42–68. Department of Health and Human Services, Rockville, MD.

Hubbard, R. L., Marsden, M. E., Rachal, J. V., *et al*. (1989). *Drug abuse treatment: a national study of effectiveness*. University of North Carolina Press, Chapel Hill.

Newcombe, R. (1992). The reduction of drug-related harm. A conceptual framework for theory, practice and research. In *The reduction of drug related harm* (ed. P. O'Hare, R. Newcombe, A. Matthews, E. Buning, E. Drucker), pp. 1–14. Routledge, London.

Preble, E. and Miller, T. (1977). Methadone, wine and welfare. In *Street ethnography* (ed. R. S. Weppner), pp. 229–48. Sage Publications, Beverley Hills, CA.

Stimson, G. (1990). Revising policy and practice: new ideas about the drugs problem. In *AIDS and drug misuse: the challenge for policy and practice in the 1990s* (ed. J. Strang and G. Stimson), pp. 121–31. Routledge, London.

Strang, J. (1990). Intermediate goals and the process of change. In *AIDS and drug misuse: The challenge for policy and practice in the 1990s* (ed. J. Strang and G. Stimson), pp. 211–21. Routledge, London.

Strang, J. and Farrell, M. (1992). Harm minimisation for drug users: when second best may be best first. *British Medical Journal*, **304**, 1127–8.

Strang, J., Heathcote, S., and Watson, P. (1987). Habit moderation in injecting addicts. *Health Trends*, **19**, 16–18.

Strang, J., Des Jarlais, D. C., Griffiths, P., and Gossop, M. (1992). The study of transitions in the route of drug use: the route from one route to another. *British Journal of Addiction*, **87**, 473–84.

Strang, J., Seivewright, N., and Farrell, M. (1993). Oral and intravenous abuse of benzodiazepines. In *Benzodiazepines dependence* (ed. C. Hallstrom), pp. 128–42. Oxford University Press, Oxford.

Winick, C. (1962). Maturing out of narcotic addiction. *Bulletin of Narcotics*, **142**, 1–7.

13

Change in the addictions: does treatment make a difference? What smoking research can tell

MARTIN JARVIS

INTRODUCTION

Those of us who earn our crust by researching and providing treatment for substance users have much to be modest about. It is not that large numbers of drinkers, smokers, and drug users do not give up. Addicts certainly do change, but this frequently appears to have little to do with the process of treatment (Wille 1978; Vaillant 1983; Chapman 1986; Klingemann 1991; Willms 1991). We all too often fail to attract clients into treatment, and when we do the typical outcome is relapse to continued drug use. This is equally the case whether we are talking about alcohol, illicit drugs, or tobacco. We console ourselves with the thought that we are addressing chronic relapsing conditions which run their course over many years. This is true, but it is also true that we have found it hard to develop treatments with demonstrable specific efficacy. One commentator, sympathetic to our cause, but also aware of the complexity of the change process, recently wrote that treatment is 'at best a timely nudge or whisper in a long life course' (Edwards 1989). Others, less charitable, have talked about treatments, for smoking at any rate, as being 'trivial interventions' and 'in the worst traditions of inconsequential research' (Chapman 1986).

The task of this chapter is to consider what implications the processes of change in addictive behaviours have for the provision of treatments. This author is aware both of the limitations of his knowledge when it comes to treatment for alcohol and illicit drugs, and of the very different considerations which apply with these substances as opposed to tobacco. Factors other than those which stem from the change process and which influence the provision of treatment include the following: the prevalence of use and the acute social harm it occasions; referrals from the legal system; collateral threats to public health (for example drugs and HIV); and associated psychiatric morbidity. In all of these respects tobacco stands out as being quite different. Tobacco is a largely invisible drug in that it causes little acute social disruption and is not particularly associated with psychopathology. Perhaps as a result, little if any public money is spent on treatment programmes for tobacco smokers, while alcohol and drug units are a familiar part of the NHS scene. In the USA an estimated $1.6 billion was spent on State-provided treatment for alcohol and other drug abuse in 1988 (Butynski 1991). Comparable figures for expenditure on treatment facilities for tobacco smoking are not available, no doubt because such programmes are conspicuous by their absence.

Issues concerning the treatment of tobacco smokers are, therefore, in many ways distinct from those relating to alcohol and drug use. The overriding question for tobacco is whether treatment should be provided at all, or whether policy should rather focus on measures which increase smokers' desire to stop (price, health education campaigns, restrictions on smoking in public places, advertising bans, etc.), and leave them to get on with the actual stopping by themselves. More subtle questions of how treatment can be made to mesh productively with the cycle of change can only be addressed when this prior matter is resolved.

Discussion in this chapter will be largely limited to tobacco. It will focus first on the broad question of the justification for treatment to help tobacco smokers stop, and then briefly how such treatment should be delivered and targeted to best effect.

SMOKING: A SUITABLE CASE FOR TREATMENT?

Because smoking is amenable to study by survey techniques, quite a bit is known about patterns of use and the smoker's career. The typical smoker takes up the habit in adolescence and continues to smoke until aged 60 or older. Some 70 per cent of adult smokers report ever having stopped for at least a week, but in nearly a half that period of abstinence lasted for less than a month and in two-thirds was longer than a year ago (NOP 1992). Dependent patterns of smoking are the norm, with less than 10 per cent of cigarette smokers in the general population being true light or occasional cigarette smokers of less than 5 cigarettes per day (OPCS 1990). Among male smokers average consumption is 17 cigarettes per day, and among women 14. Over half of all smokers light up their first cigarette of the day within 30 minutes of waking (NOP 1992). Most smokers in the UK appear to want to quit: in a recent survey two-thirds of both heavy and light smokers answered 'yes' to the question 'Do you want to give up smoking altogether?' and the majority stated that their desire to quit was strong. However, of those who wanted to give up, only 13 per cent (15 per cent of light smokers and 8 per cent of heavy) thought they would be very likely to succeed if they decided to give up in the next 3 months (NOP 1992).

The picture that emerges from this assortment of facts is that dependence on tobacco is not confined to a minority of users, but is rather the norm. That dependence is not, of course, an all-or-none phenomenon, but graded in extent. Nevertheless, it would appear to be a significant problem for at least 7 million smokers in the United Kingdom.

If what smokers say can be taken at face value, a comfortable majority want to stop, and indeed have made a number of attempts to do so. They continue to smoke mainly because not smoking is difficult. On the face of it, this would seem to imply that offering them some help would not be a bad idea.

PATTERNS OF CESSATION

The prevalence of smoking has declined markedly in the past two decades. Some of this is due to reductions in recruitment, but a major part reflects quitting. There are now some 10–11 million ex-smokers in Britain, and an estimated 1.3 million new ex-smokers each year in the USA. In both countries the vast majority (90 per cent or more) have succeeded without recourse to any formal treatment. In terms of population cessation rates (that is ex-smokers as a percentage of ever-regular smokers), we have gone in Britain from 21 per cent in 1973 to 40 per cent in 1988 (Jarvis and Jackson 1988; OPCS 1990). While this is encouraging, some observers might be less than overwhelmingly impressed, pointing to both the fact that even now only 40 per cent succeed in becoming ex-smokers by the age of 60, and to the wide disparity in cessation rates by social class: 56 per cent in professional but only 30 per cent in unskilled working groups (OPCS 1990).

THE ARGUMENT AGAINST SMOKING CESSATION TREATMENT

Schachter (1982) was the first to stir controversy when he claimed that smoking was not the recalcitrant condition many supposed. He interviewed colleagues at Columbia University and residents of a small Long Island town and found that 64 per cent of those who had attempted to quit smoking had succeeded, for an average of 7.4 years. He contrasted this with the typical 10–25 per cent one-year outcome of therapeutic interventions with clinical populations, and concluded that the explanation for the difference 'must be either in the perversity of those who seek help, or alternatively in terms of the perversity of the therapeutic process proper'.

A further onslaught on the value of intensive treatments for smokers came from Chapman (1985) in a piece provocatively titled 'Stop-smoking clinics: a case for their abandonment'. Chapman referred to Raw and Heller's survey (1984), which indicated that the 55 stop-smoking clinics in the UK might help a total of less than 2000 people to stop smoking in a year, or only 1 in every 5000 smokers currently wanting to stop— an 'utterly insignificant contribution'.

The offence of smoking clinics was compounded by their claimed counterproductive effects on the public's attitudes:

There is the expectation that stopping is extremely difficult and that one should place oneself passively in the hands of a healer... Provision of cessation clinics and groups perpetuates the idea that smoking has to be cured, so inhibiting the growth of confidence in self-directed cessation.

Nor would he allow that clinics met the needs of a particular hard core of heavily dependent smokers, claiming that there was no evidence that clinic attenders differed from self-quitters in terms of smoking habit, smoking history, number of attempts to stop, or personality.

Just one exception was granted to the general rule of the uselessness of treatment. This was the value of GPs' contact with smokers in their everyday practice, as exemplified by Russell's study (Russell *et al.* 1979) which indicated that the yield from brief advice routinely delivered could amount to half a million ex-smokers a year across the whole country.

THE DEFENCE

Critics have challenged a number of aspects of Schachter's and Chapman's arguments. There are obvious problems of a small and biased sample in Schachter's study (Jeffrey and Wing, 1983), and it has been convincingly demonstrated that the success rates of single self-initiated quit attempts are in fact considerably lower than from clinic interventions (Cohen *et al.* 1989). It has also become apparent that clinic attenders are indeed more dependent than the general population of smokers (Fiore *et al.* 1990).

But Chapman's core point is well taken: from a public health perspective, clinic interventions risk irrelevance if they can only address the needs of a tiny minority and at an unacceptable cost.

IS GP ADVICE ENOUGH?

In view of the minimal resources invested in smoking clinics, Chapman's assault on them smacks of overkill. But is his alternative of an approach which combines active smoking control measures by governments with routine advice by health professionals in primary care sufficient? The cost−efficacy of an intervention which yields a long-term success rate of 5 per cent for only 2 or 3 minutes face-to-face contact is apparent, but it is not immediately clear whether this is the best that can be done to meet smokers' needs. To examine this further, analyses have been carried out on the relationship of pretreatment subject measures to outcome in the Russell study.

Russell *et al.*'s (1979) sample comprised all cigarette smokers attending their GP for whatever reason over a two-week period. It was thus a reasonably unbiased sample of the general smoking population. Subjects were randomized to four conditions: non-intervention controls, questionnaire-only controls, advice only, and advice and warning of follow-up. Long-term success, defined as abstinence from smoking at both one-month and one-year follow-up was 0.3, 1.6, 3.3 and 5.1 per cent, respectively in the four conditions.

Prior to seeing the doctor, subjects in three of the groups completed a questionnaire covering smoking and personal details. Responses to this questionnaire have been factor analysed, yielding the 4-factor solution shown in Table 13.1. The factors are easily identifiable as Dependence, Motivation, Drinking behaviour, and Smoking environment.

To consider the way scores on these factors relate to outcome, subjects were divided into four groups varying along the dimension of whether they attempted to quit smoking, and how long the quit-attempt lasted. Assigned treatment condition is ignored in this classification. The derivation of the four groups is given in Table 13.2.

Scores on all four factors were significantly related to the outcome classification, but only weakly so in the case of 'Smoking environment'

TABLE 13.1 *Four factor solution to pretreatment questionnaire responses in Russell* et al. *study (1979)*

Category	Loading
1. Dependence	
How difficult would you find it to go without smoking for as long as one week?	0.88
If you decided to give up smoking completely **in the next three weeks**, how likely do you think you would be to succeed?	0.81
On occasions when you can't smoke or you haven't got any cigarettes on you, do you feel a craving for one?	0.80
When you smoke, about how many cigarettes do you usually smoke in a day?	0.73
2. Motivation	
Do you have any intention of giving up smoking completely **in the next three weeks**?	0.77
How much do you want to stop smoking?	0.78
About how many times have you tried to give up smoking altogether?	0.72
3. Drinking behaviour	
About how often, on average, have you had an alcoholic drink over the past year?	0.91
About how often, on average, have you been to a pub or bar over the past year?	0.91
4. Smoking environment	
About how many of your friends are smokers?	0.75
About how much of your average day is spent in the company of smokers?	0.72
Is your husband/wife or any other person you live with a smoker?	0.59

($p < 0.05$) (see Fig 13.4). The must powerful relationships were with Motivation and Dependence. As illustrated in Fig. 13.1, Smokers scored substantially lower than the other three groups on Motivation, while the differences among the Triers, Relapsers, and Quitters did not reach significance. On Dependence (Fig. 13.2), Quitters and Relapsers scored significantly lower than Smokers and Triers, who did not differ from

TABLE 13.2 *General practice advice study: Russell* et al. *(1979)*

Smokers (*n* = 1115)	Smoking at 1 month and 1 year; no quit attempt
Triers (*n* = 255)	Smoking at 1 month and 1 year; quit attempt reported at 1 month
Relapsers (*n* = 50)	Abstinent at 1 month, smoking at 1 year
Quitters (*n* = 49)	Abstinent at 1 month and at 1 year

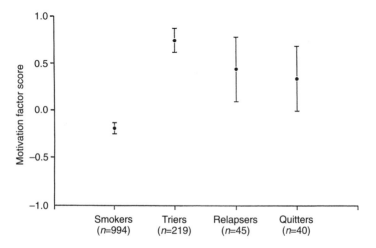

FIG. 13.1 Relation of motivation to outcome: GP advice study (after Russell *et al.* 1979). Data is shown as a mean value with 95 per cent confidence limits.

each other. On Drinking Behaviour (Fig. 13.3), the Quitters stood out from the other groups as having significantly less involvement with alcohol.

If we attempt a brief characterization of each of the outcome groups, it might be as follows:

Smokers:	low motivation,	high dependence
Triers:	high motivation,	high dependence
Relapsers:	high motivation,	medium dependence
Quitters:	high motivation,	low dependence, low drinking

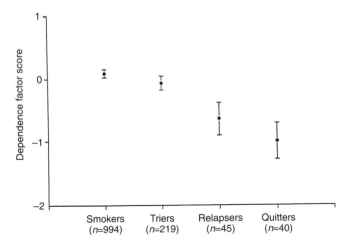

FIG. 13.2 Relation of dependence to outcome: GP advice study (after Russell *et al.* 1979). Data is shown as a mean value with 95 per cent confidence limits.

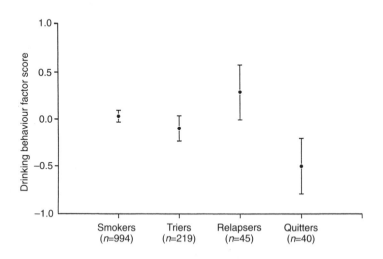

FIG. 13.3 Relation of drinking to outcome: GP advice study (after Russell *et al.* 1979). Data is shown as a mean value with 95 per cent confidence limits.

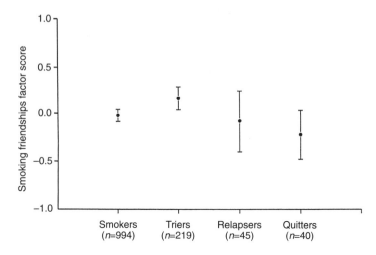

FIG. 13.4 Relation of smoking friendships to outcome: GP advice study (after Russell *et al*. 1979). Data is shown as a mean value with 95 per cent confidence limits.

In terms of stages of change theories, such as that of Prochaska and Di Clemente (1983), the Smokers would represent precontemplators, while the other three groups would all be contemplators. The effect of the intervention was to give a boost to motivation and prompt a quit attempt. For a small number of subjects, who were light, low-dependent smokers, this was sufficient to achieve long-term cessation. But for a much larger group, success was blocked by dependence, and GPs' advice did nothing to overcome this. Dependence emerges as the key construct militating against successful change. Chapman's point that only interventions that can reach the whole community have the capacity to influence national rates of smoking prevalence is well taken, but unless interventions in primary care can address the issue of dependence, they would seem likely to fall far short of their potential for achieving change.

LESSONS FROM GP ADVICE

There are a number of lessons we can learn from the Russell study. First, in the general population of smokers who are not specifically seeking help to give up tobacco, there is a substantial group who are at a point in their smoking career where they are open and potentially responsive to GP intervention. This group varies widely in dependence, however, and it is only the small minority of lightest smokers for whom simple advice is sufficient. For a much larger group dependence blocks the way to successful cessation. What appears to be needed is the incorporation, into GP interventions, of approaches which specifically address the problem of dependence.

Most smokers do not want formal treatment, and the great majority who have quit say that they did it by themselves. How do we square this with the evidence that smokers do in fact respond to GPs' intervention? One answer to this paradox may be that smokers do not consider brief advice from a GP as a treatment, even if it affects their quitting behaviour. In a recent survey of the US population (Fiore *et al.* 1990), over 90 per cent of successful quitters said that they had done so unassisted. However, 74 per cent also said that they had at some point been advised to quit by a doctor.

MAKING GP INTERVENTION MORE EFFECTIVE

There is an obvious way to attempt to improve GPs' success—namely by incorporating nicotine replacement into the treatment mix. Treatment aids which target dependence have been available for more than 10 years now. Nicotine chewing gum was first evaluated in intensive clinic settings, where it was shown to approximately double success rates over placebo when both were combined with group support and encouragement (Jarvis *et al.* 1982; Hjalmarson 1984; Lam *et al.* 1987). But in primary care settings, results have been less encouraging (Lam *et al.* 1987). The problem here appears to be one of communicating adequate instructions and expectations so as to achieve effective compliance with the use of the product. GPs all too frequently do no more than hand over a prescription without any word of explanation. As a result, patients may have quite unrealistic expectations and fail to benefit from the modest help which the gum can offer.

Despite these limitations, there is evidence that nicotine gum can function in the desired way in primary care to offset the adverse effects of increasing levels of dependence on the likelihood of successful quitting. Fig. 13.5 illustrates the results of an analysis of the predictors of outcome in a GP trial of nicotine chewing gum by Russell *et al.* (Jackson *et al.* 1986). In that study the long-term success rate in the group offered a prescription for nicotine gum, at 9 per cent, was double that of advice-only and control groups (Russell *et al.* 1983). The figure shows that, whereas in the advice and control groups higher levels of dependence were associated with markedly poorer outcome, this was

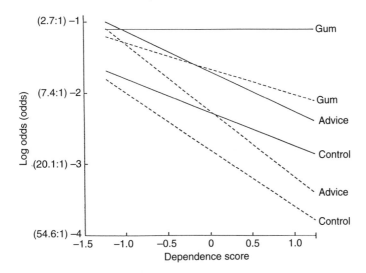

FIG. 13.5 Predictors of outcome (from Russell *et al.* in Jackson *et al.* 1986). Solid lines, male; Dashed lines, Female. The mean dependence score is zero, the standard deviation is one. The plotted lines show the predicted odds of successful quitting by level of dependence in men and women by intervention condition.

much less the case in the gum group. In men particularly, those subjects with high levels of dependence had just as good an outcome as low-dependent subjects.

There is now a mood of optimism in the air about nicotine replacement as a treatment strategy. Studies of nicotine chewing gum established the basic efficacy of this approach, and now a new range of delivery systems is under development, including nicotine skin patches (Tonnesen *et al.* 1991; Transdermal Nicotine Study Group 1991) and a nasal nicotine spray (Jarvis *et al.* 1987), which promise to address some of the limitations of nicotine gum. Nicotine skin patches seem particularly suited to primary care in that they require little explanation, and it may prove much easier than with the gum to achieve compliance with appropriate use. Published clinical trials have given good evidence of efficacy, and there are indications that intensive psychological support is not necessary to achieve good results (Abelin *et al.* 1989; Tonnesen *et al.* 1991) Recently published trials of skin patches conducted in primary care show a doubling of successful cessation over placebo both at 3 months (ICRF General Practice Research Group 1993) and one-year follow-up (Russell *et al.* 1993).

DO WE NEED INTENSIVE CLINICS AS WELL AS
INTERVENTION IN PRIMARY CARE?

If the argument so far is accepted, not only is it justified to provide treatment for smokers, it would be negligent not to do so. The evidence is clear that many smokers, perhaps a majority, are sufficiently dependent to need help; we have available treatments of demonstrated efficacy, both to stir smokers into making a cessation attempt and to make the likelihood of that attempt succeeding more probable. Treatment should be seen as the natural and necessary complement to those other arms of smoking policy which seek to educate and inform smokers and to restrict tobacco usage through the price mechanism and through availability.

Given the extent of smoking prevalence and the disinclination of smokers to see their habit as a disorder requiring specialized medical attention, the conclusion that smoking treatment has to be made a part of the routine of primary care is inescapable. No other part of our health care system has the capacity to reach all parts of the community. But is there a case to be made for having specialized clinics for smokers as well?

Chapman's argument against smokers' clinics was firstly that they could never make any sort of impact on national smoking prevalence, and secondly that they did not cater for a specially dependent subgroup. He is almost certainly right on the first point, but wrong on the second. Nevertheless, the case for clinics does not simply rest on the proposition that society should show a caring face.

Smokers clinics have never been an established part of the NHS, but could become so in the future. It has been suggested that they could justify their existence first by acting as a local centre of expertise, mobilizing and supplying GPs with intervention materials, and accepting referrals of difficult cases. The potential value of this role has been demonstrated in field research which closely linked the smokers' clinic with coordinated interventions in primary care in the local community (Russell *et al*. 1987; 1988). Secondly, they could continue to advance treatment by researching interventions with a capacity for wider implementation. Such research can only be carried out in settings where there is a steady and continuous throughput of dependent smokers. Finally, it is conceivable that one day in some distant and optimistic future, when smoking prevalence is much lower than it is now, that cigarette smoking has achieved a deviancy label similar to that now attached to alcoholism and illicit drug use, and our treatments have made such considerable advances in efficacy, that clinics will be recognized as a worthwhile response to a major social problem, as alcohol and drug units are now.

GETTING SMOKERS TO STOP OR PREVENTING RELAPSE?

The discussion so far has been entirely in terms of treatment as something which gets people to stop smoking. In view of the ubiquity of relapse, for many people this is missing the mark. The problem of giving up smoking, they say, is not stopping, but staying stopped. The numbers lend support to this view: even with state-of-the-art treatment a majority of those who initially quit subsequently relapse. This argument rapidly leads to the conclusion that, in terms of stages of change, we should be directing our efforts mainly at reducing the rate of long-term relapse, rather than seeking to increase the proportion of smokers who initially quit in response to an intervention. It is certainly true that if we could reduce the rate of relapse by even a modest amount, it would have a substantial impact on long-term cessation rates. But before recommending relapse-prevention as a policy initiative in the area of treatment, two major questions have to be addressed: is it effective, and is it cost-effective? For both the answer at present must be no.

The literature on trials of relapse prevention in smoking is rather scanty, with many of the investigations that have been published suffering from small sample sizes and low statistical power. One or two studies have hinted at possible effects, but the value of these approaches has not been clearly established (Hall *et al.* 1984; Stevens and Hollis 1989). The largest single study was of the MRFIT cohort, in which 8194 cigarette smokers were randomized to a Special Intervention group (SI) or Usual Care (UC). Men in the SI group received an initial highly intensive 10-week smoking intervention, and then entered a maintenance or extended intervention programme depending on whether they had achieved abstinence. Despite this, only two-thirds of those who reported not smoking at one-year follow-up maintained abstinence up to four years (Ockene *et al.* 1982). Seven per cent and five per cent of subjects stopped for the first time in years 2 and 3, but about 40 per cent in each case had relapsed again by the following year. Only 8 per cent of those who were abstinent at the four-year point were relapsers who had stopped again. Set against the very large investment of resources in extended treatment, these outcomes look disappointing.

Relapse prevention must for the present be regarded as a promising idea needing further research development, rather than a treatment ripe for implementation. We should perhaps acknowledge that many who initially quit will relapse. But they are not lost, and can return for a further episode of treatment when they feel ready for it.

ACCELERATING THE DECLINE IN TOBACCO PREVALENCE: THE NEED FOR TREATMENT

In 1987 the WHO Regional Committee for Europe adopted an ambitious plan which envisaged a 50 per cent reduction in tobacco consumption, and smoking prevalence in all countries of no more than 20 per cent by 1995. They have recently had to acknowledge that these objectives will not be met (WHO Tobacco Alert 1992). However, both the USA and the UK have now set even more ambitious goals for the year 2000. In the USA the target prevalence is 15 per cent (US Public Health Service 1989), and in the UK a figure of 20 per cent has been adopted in the *Health of the Nation* targets (Secretary of State for Health 1991).

Reaching these goals will not be easy. Reducing the uptake of smoking by adolescents has proved difficult, and in any event would have only a minor impact. The main burden will fall on improving cessation rates. It has been estimated that there will need to be a 50 per cent increase in the current population cessation rate, from some 42 to 63 per cent, if the UK targets are to be met (Jarvis and Russell, 1991), and the prospects for the USA will be at least as demanding (Pierce *et al*. 1989 *a*, *b*). Given the addictive nature of the smoking habit, it seems unlikely that current policies alone will be sufficient. These considerations for the future reinforce earlier arguments based on factors influencing change in smokers in suggesting that widespread application of treatment is urgently needed.

CONCLUSIONS

This paper has focused on tobacco in considering the implications of the change process for treatment. Priorities for interventions in alcohol and drug use may be different, but at least one common theme may be the need to channel treatment through primary care so as to reach the general population of users, rather than just a highly selected minority (Wallace *et al*. 1988; Saunders 1989).

Nicotine dependence appears to lie at the heart of the difficulties smokers experience in quitting. The majority of smokers in the population experience a significant degree of dependence, and it is this rather than lack of motivation which seems to be the main stumbling block to faster rates of decline in national smoking prevalence. A small proportion of smokers respond to a simple motivational input, but a much greater number need help to overcome their dependence.

Research over the past decade has shown the efficacy of nicotine replacement as a treatment approach, and new developments such as the nicotine skin patch may be particularly suited to application in primary care. Treatment for smokers is certainly needed, and if adopted by the health care system, could make a significant impact on improving the nation's health.

REFERENCES

Abelin, T., Buehler, A., Müller, P., Vesanen, K., and Imhoff, P. R. (1989). Controlled trial of transdermal nicotine patch in tobacco withdrawal. *Lancet*, i, 7–10.

Butynski, W. (1991). Drug treatment services: Funding and admissions. In *Improving drug abuse treatment* (ed. R. W. Pickens, D. S. W. Leukefeld, and C. R. Schuster), pp. 20–52. NIDA Research Monograph, No 106. USDHHS, Washington DC.

Chapman, S. (1985). Stop-smoking clinics: a case for their abandonment. *Lancet*, i, 918–20.

Chapman, S. (1986). The natural history of smoking cessation: How and why people stop smoking. Health Education Council, London.

Cohen, S., Lichtenstein, E., Prochaska, J. O., *et al*. (1989). Debunking myths about self-quitting: evidence from 10 prospective studies of persons quitting smoking by themselves. *American Psychologist*, 44, 1355–65.

Edwards, G. E. (1989). As the years go rolling by: Drinking problems in the time dimension. *British Journal of Psychiatry*, 154, 18–26.

Fiore, M. C., Novotny, T. E., Pierce, J. P., *et al*. (1990). Methods used to quit smoking in the United States: Do cessation programs help? *Journal of the American Medical Association*, 263, 2760–5.

Hall, S. M., Tunstall, C., Rugg, D., and Jones, R. T. (1984). Preventing relapse to smoking by behavioral skills training. *Journal of Consulting and Clinical Psychology*, 52, 372–8.

Hjalmarson, A. I. M. (1984). Effect of nicotine chewing gum in smoking cessation: a randomized placebo-controlled, double blind study. *Journal of the American Medical Association*, 252, 2835–48.

Imperial Cancer Research Fund General Practice Research Group (1993). Effectiveness of a nicotine patch in helping people stop smoking: results of a randomised trial in general practice. *British Medical Journal*, 306, 1304–8.

Jackson, P. H., Stapleton, J. A., Russell, M. A. H., and Merriman, R. J. (1986). Predictors of outcome in a general practitioner intervention against smoking. *Preventive Medicine*, 15, 244–53.

Jarvis, M. J. and Jackson, P. H. (1988). Cigar and pipe smoking in Britain:

implications for smoking prevalence and cessation. *British Journal of Addiction*, **83**, 323–30.

Jarvis, M. J. and Russell, M. A. H. (1991). Smoking targets for the year 2000. Evidence submitted to the Department of Health in response to the *Health of the Nation* Green Paper, October 1991.

Jarvis, M. J., Raw, M., Russell, M. A. H., and Feyerabend, C. (1982). Randomised controlled trial of nicotine chewing gum. *British Medical Journal*, **285**, 537–40.

Jarvis, M. J., Hajek, P., Russell, M. A. H., West, R. J., and Feyerabend, C. (1987). Nasal nicotine solution as an aid to cigarette withdrawal: a pilot clinical trial. *British Journal of Addiction*, **82**, 983–8.

Jeffrey, R. W. and Wing, R. R. (1983). Recidivism and self-cure of smoking and obesity: Data from population studies. *American Psychologist*, **38**, 852.

Klingemann, H. K. H. (1991). The motivation for change from problem alcohol and heroin use. *British Journal of Addiction*, **86**, 727–44.

Lam, W., Sze, P. C., Sacks, H. S., and Chalmers, T. C. (1987). Meta-analysis of randomised controlled trials of nicotine chewing gum. *Lancet*, **ii**, 27–9.

NOP Omnibus Services. (1992). *Smoking habits 1991: Research carried out for the Department of Health*. Department of Health, London.

Ockene, J. K., Hymowitz, N., Sexton, M., and Broste, S. K. (1982). Comparison of patterns of smoking behavior change among smokers in the Multiple Risk Intervention Trial (MRFIT) *Preventive Medicine*, **11**, 621–38.

Office of Population Censuses and Surveys. (1990). *General Household Survey, 1988*. HMSO, London.

Pierce, J. P., Fiore, M. C., Novotny, T. E., Hatziandreu, E. J., and Davis, R. M. (1989*a*). Trends in cigarette smoking in the United States: Projections to the year 2000. *Journal of the American Medical Association*, **261**, 61–5.

Pierce, J. P., Fiore, M. C., Novotny, T. E., Hatziandreu, E. J., and Davis, R. M. (1989*b*). Trends in cigarette smoking in the United States: Educational differences are increasing. *Journal of the American Medical Association*, **261**, 56–60.

Prochaska, J. O. and Di Clemente, C. C. (1983). Stages and processes of self-change of smoking: Towards an integrative model of change. *Journal of Consulting and Clinical Psychology*, **51**, 390–5.

Raw, M. and Heller J. (1984). *Helping people to stop smoking. The development, role and potential of support services in the UK*. Health Education Council, London.

Russell, M. A. H., Wilson, C., Taylor, C., and Baker, C. D. (1979). Effect of general practitioners' advice against smoking. *British Medical Journal*, **2**, 231–5.

Russell, M. A. H., Merriman, R., Stapleton, J. A., and Taylor, W. (1983). Effect of nicotine chewing gum as an adjunct to general practitioners' advice against smoking. *British Medical Journal*, **287**, 1782–5.

Russell, M. A. H., Stapleton, J. A., Jackson, P. H., Hajek, P., and Feyerabend, C. (1987). District programme to reduce smoking: effect of clinic supported brief intervention by general practitioners. *British Medical Journal*, **295**, 1240–4.

Russell, M. A. H., Stapleton, J. A., Hajek, P., Jackson, P. H., and Feyerabend, C. (1988). District programme to reduce smoking: can sustained intervention by general practitioners affect prevalence? *Journal of Epidemiology Community Health*, **42**, 111–15.

Russell, M. A. H., Stapleton, J. A., Feyerabend, C., Wiseman, S. M., Gustavsson, G., Sawe, U., and Connor, P. (1993). Targeting heavy smokers in general practice: randomised controlled trial of transdermal nicotine patches. *British Medical Journal*, **306**, 1308–12.

Saunders, J. B. (1989). The efficacy of treatment for drinking problems. *International Review of Psychiatry*, **1**, 121–38.

Schachter, S. (1982). Recidivism and self-cure of smoking and obesity. *American Psychologist*, **37**, 436–44.

Secretary of State for Health. (1992). *The health of the nation*, (Cm 1986). HMSO, London.

Stevens, V. J. and Hollis, J. F. (1989). Preventing smoking relapse, using an individually tailored skills-training technique. *Journal of Consulting and Clinical Psychology*, **57**, 420–4.

Tonnesen, P., Norregaard, J., Simonsen, K., and Sawe, U. (1991). A double-blind trial of a 16-hour transdermal nicotine patch in smoking cessation. *New England Journal of Medicine*, **325**, 311–15.

Transdermal Nicotine Study Group. (1991). Transdermal nicotine for smoking cessation: six-month results from two multicenter controlled clinical trials. *Journal of the American Medical Association*, **266**, 3133–8.

US Public Health Service. (1989). *Promoting health/preventing disease: Year 2000 objectives for the nation*. US Department of Health and Human Services, Public Health Service, Washington DC.

Vaillant, G. E. (1983). *The natural history of alcoholism*. Harvard University Press, Cambridge MA.

Wallace, P., Cutler, S., and Haines, A. (1988). Randomized controlled trial of general practitioner intervention in patients with excessive alcohol consumption. *British Medical Journal*, **297**, 663–8.

WHO (1992). *Tobacco alert*. WHO, Geneva.

Wille, R. (1978). Cessation of opiate dependence: processes involved in achieving abstinence. *British Journal of Addiction*, **73**, 381–4.

Willms, D. G. (1991). A new stage, a new life: individual success in quitting smoking. *Social Science and Medicine*, **33**, 1365–71.

14

Technical habiliments, science, and the clinical frontline: asking some questions

GRIFFITH EDWARDS

The purpose of this final chapter is to explore the possibility of further bridgings between the scientific analyses of individual change processes presented earlier in this book, and the awkward problems of human behaviour as encountered at the clinical frontline. The task is made easier by the fact that authors who write from a theoretical perspective about the treatment of substance dependence are usually also themselves clinical practitioners: there is no great divide between scientists and journeymen. Thomas Trotter, in one of the earliest treatises to discuss change processes and drinking problems, cautioned, however, thus:

The practice of physic is sometimes so tightly laced in technical habiliments that it is incapable of turning around.

(Trotter 1804).

This book is not intended as a clinical handbook, and it would be too great a demand to expect it to provide instant answers on how to treat the next patient who presents at tomorrow's clinic. Nonetheless, it would have failed in its intentions if it did not address the clinical world, and examine the relevance of science to what is said and done in tomorrow's clinic. Science can, though, itself often become too tight laced, too bound up in theories, and too focused on its own predilections, and the scientists will benefit by being repeatedly challenged by the painful, disorderly, complexities of the clinical world. Science in this area sometimes seems to operate in terms of a distinctly sanitized version of the human condition. The trade in probing questions should, therefore, not be just one way.

This chapter will be structured around three areas of questioning which might usefully be explored if science and clinical practice are to communicate in a two-way fashion on the understanding and actualization of individual change in substance-seeking behaviour. The three areas which will be sequentially considered in this bridging fashion will firstly be the relevance of relapse prevention strategies to the generality of clinical practice. The second area for debate will be the psychology of motivation. If relapse prevention and motivation represent two cutting-edge concerns for the relationship between science and clinical practice in this arena, the third topic which has been selected for attention is not one which currently attracts many headlines. The focus under this third heading will be on the understanding of why some patients, despite our best efforts, get worse.

The purpose of this chapter is thus that of identifying questions rather than promulgation of any fixed or final answers. The three topics selected for debate are chosen somewhat arbitrarily from the much larger array of questions raised in this book, in other books, in every clinical encounter, and in the deep nights of our own doubts, and which together bear on how the scientific and clinical worlds are to be better bridged.

In passing, one might do well to take cognizance of the following highly relevant passage which is to be found in a text written by a distinguished Victorian physician, and which is taken from a chapter which dealt with 'Disease from errors of dress' (Richardson 1883).

At one time a widespread and very dangerous disease was induced in women by one particular error of dress, the error of lacing up the body, tightly, in stays. The disease was sometimes fatal... In these days some improvement has taken place in respect to tight lacing of the body, but the evil is not altogether removed.

Even today we would do well to avoid a too tight lacing of technical habiliments, lest the outcome be fatal to true advance.

HOW USEFUL ARE RELAPSE PREVENTION STRATEGIES IN THE GENERALITY OF CLINICAL PRACTICE?

The theoretical basis for relapse prevention has been discussed by Robin Davidson in Chapter 4 of this book. One does well to remember that the term does not imply a single theory or just one intervention technique, but the deployment of a range of methods deriving from a variety of behavioural and cognitive postulates. There are controlled trials to show that when such techniques are applied to certain patient groups, these kinds of approach can offer significant therapeutic gain (Stitzer *et al.* 1983; Marlatt and Gordon 1985; Miller and Hester 1986; Saunders 1989; Bien *et al.* 1993). No therapeutic intervention is ever likely to generalize in its utility to the total potential patient population, and it would be unfair to put this expectation upon relapse prevention. Behavioural treatment may be more effective with some substances than with others, and it is probably not very efficacious with cigarette smoking (Jarvis and Russell 1989). The question of the degree of generalizability should therefore be addressed, and has not yet received adequate attention. In raising these and other questions about relapse prevention, one is attempting further to explore the connection between the research and clinical domains, without in any way casting doubt on the value of an approach which reminds us that dependence is best seen not as mysterious enchantment but rationally as learnt habit. Again, to quote Trotter:

The habit of drunkenness is a disease of the mind. The soul itself has received impressions that are incompatible with its reasoning powers.

Provisionally, some of the relevant issues within this area can be identified as follows:

1. *Treatment uptake*. From among the next hundred patients enrolling at a drug dependence or alcohol problems clinic, what percentage will be able to benefit from formal application of a relapse prevention approach? The therapeutic past is littered with parallel examples where the reflex answer of 'everyone' was given—everyone for group therapy, everyone a suitable case for AA, absolutely everyone for antabuse. A therapeutic approach has in reality only come of age when the criteria for its application have been parsimoniously defined. Exclusion criteria which militate against the application of relapse prevention techniques need to be more sharply articulated.

2. *Is it possible usefully to conduct relapse prevention therapies with patients who are maintained on a therapeutic psychoactive drug, or who are repeatedly revisiting alcohol or other drugs*? In the general field of behaviour therapy and particularly in relation to the treatment of phobic states, there has been debate as to whether psychological treatments can profitably be employed when a patient is being given a benzodiazepine or any other type of anxiolytic drug. There are arguments which suggest that the chemical dampening of anxiety can interfere with the psychological processes inherent in desensitization: anxiety cannot be extinguished when it is not being aroused (Gray 1987). Within

that perspective one might not only want to consider the relevance of, say, methadone or an antidepressant with sedative properties to the application of a relapse prevention technique, but also the influence on learning processes of the psychological cover given by disulfiram or naltrexone. There is no reason to assume an inevitable antipathy between behavioural and psychopharmacological treatments, and some recent research has elegantly demonstrated the possibility of synergistic effects (O'Malley *et al.* 1992). But to leave the benefits of psycho-pharmacology or the cross-cutting complications of continued or inter-mittent use of heroin, cocaine, or alcohol out of the reckoning when discussing the application of psychological treatments in this field of practice, is to close out a large part of reality. The seminal research on the behaviour therapy of phobic states (Freeman and Kendrick 1960), or obsessional disorder (Rachman and Hodgson 1980), was not done with patients who binged on alcohol or cocaine.

3. *The abstinence violation effect.* It is argued by champions of the relapse prevention approach that setting up the expectation that the taking of one drink will inevitably result in a precipitous slide into the pit of full relapse, will encourage the person who takes that one drink to let go and slide—hence the abstinence violation effect (Marlatt and Gordon 1985). The relapse prevention therapist is not blasé about relapse, but will be likely to convey to the patient a message that relapse, if it occurs, is something to be learnt from and intelligently analysed, rather than a fearsome and unmitigated disaster. To what extent is that approach compatible with the Alcoholics Anonymous or Narcotics Anonymous philosophies? Given the wide prevalence of AA and NA as a helping resource and the now considerable influence of relapse prevention, it would be a pity if the two approaches were to come to be seen as irreconcilable because of dispute over one narrow issue. In reality, the dispute is probably more imagined than real. There is little research evidence to show that an abstinence violation effect exists (Birke *et al.* 1990; O'Malley *et al.* 1992), and AA teaching and relapse prevention strategies share much common ground. But again to quote Thomas Trotter (a compulsive habit perhaps), we would be foolish to ignore the fact that alcohol can be an immensely powerful *cue* for further alcohol seeking behaviour:

As soon as the limited portion of liquor is swallowed, an agreeable glow is experienced; and by it so grateful a feeling is conveyed to the mind, which in an instant connects the chain of habit, that is our duty to break ... as he is aware that the effect of the present dose will only be of short duration, he must take another to prolong his reverie, and ward off some intruding care. With a second glass he finds more pleasing objects presented to his imagination, and then he is urged to try a third ... and he goes on, libation after libation, till he sinks into a drunken slumber.

There is merit in learning how to deal with relapse, but for the dependent patient greater merit still in learning how to avoid relapse and break the chain of habit.

4. *Therapy, periphery, and centrally.* At worst and clumsily applied, relapse prevention concentrates on little hits of peripheral behaviour while ignoring the centrality of the patient's existential reality. The nurse sits in a corner completing a relapse prevention matrix with the patient, carefully plans and sets up a programme of practice for cue exposure, talks through a repertoire of coping skills, identifies and warns against dangerous situations, but ignores the fact that this patient deeply cannot conceive of the possibility for change, sees him or herself as scripted for self-destruction, perceives the world as hostile, and those who offer help as untrustworthy. To engage in a mere re-run of old conflictual debates between behavioural and dynamic therapies, would be unprofitable. If, however, a treatment facility rather than adopting relapse prevention as a part of a total therapeutic armentarium makes of these useful methods not technique but a total and exclusive institutional philosophy, that institution will teach tricks, but not in any real sense offer healing (Miller 1989).

HOW IS MOTIVATION TO BE WON OR MADE?

Psychological theories on motivation for personal change have been considered at several points in this book, particularly in Chapters 4, 6, and 7. Motivational interviewing as a therapeutic technique has over recent years attracted considerable attention (Miller and Rollnick 1991), and without doubt the last few years have seen the development of useful psychological input into ideas on how motivation is to be enhanced in the clinical setting. The concept of motivation as an all-or-none state, the nihilistic segmentation of patients into those who are 'motivated' or alternatively 'unmotivated', the view of motivation as a commodity which the patient brings with him or her and about which nothing much can be done, all this is being replaced by a more subtle and dynamic formulation of motivation as complex, dimensional, and malleable (Prochaska and DiClemente 1983; Saunders and Wilkinson 1990; Klingemann 1991, and see Chapter 6). Around this topic the following questions can arise at the clinical frontline.

1. *How significant to recovery is the road to Damascus*? Both clinical experience and research literature testify to the existence of recoveries which appear to have come about in response to acute or cataclysmic events which are seen by the individual as having provided an intensely meaningful and personal turning point (Tuchfeld 1981; Vaillant 1983; Ludwig 1985). A recent research report (Edwards *et al.* 1992) quoted the following case instance:

Subject. 'I was reading a magazine one day, an Irish paper. They were advertising for a place in Ireland called Knock where the Virgin appeared. I was quite interested. And I sent a donation, got friendly with the parish priest, terribly interested in the apparition there, you know, and it's all gone from there. I attribute everything to that particular place. I visited the place, atmosphere, and I just knew I would never drink again or smoke. But as I say, I'm not a religious nutter.'

Interviewer. 'Did the change come gradually. Did you see it as a sudden change?'

Subject. 'I think I changed overnight. I honestly, truthfully do, I think that's how it happened. I didn't have any flash of light, I never thought I saw God. It happened. And that's all I can tell you. It happened, why question it?'

Before dismissing such case histories as rare or merely exotic, one should consider the possibility that although the incidence of such occurrences will be low within the duration of any single 12-month follow-up series, their relevance may be considerably more significant as judged within the time frame of a drinking career. It can, of course, also fairly be argued that what appears to be a sudden change is much more probably only the outward manifestation of a prolonged and preliminary preparation for that breakpoint in behaviour (Sobell *et al.* 1993). Furthermore, the cataclysmic turning points which are memorable because they mark true and lasting change, are in reality likely to be matched by many equally dramatic 'turning points' which proved to be only ephemeral, and which are then conveniently forgotten.

With those provisoes entered, one may still ask whether the Damascus type of event can speak to an important aspect of the change process which is not at present sufficiently captured in academic formulations, nor sufficiently exploited for therapeutic ends. Manifestly it is none too easy to create miracles to order, and most therapists would be uncomfortable if asked to take on the role of miracle worker, although such practice was an essential part of the shaman's job. We should though perhaps be more willing to admit that radical shifts in belief and behaviour are a human possibility, and be more willing to encourage our patients to prepare for, and to be open to, the possibility of such existential experience.

2. *Motivation to change and the rewards of life.* Looked at in the long term, patients seem often to consolidate their recovery because for them being sober has become more rewarding than continuing with drink or drugs. The patient has not performed the formal calculations, but there is the live sense of the pay-off from the decision-making matrix being weighted toward sobriety, and with a calculus of positive outcomes which would now be unthinkable to throw away (Orford 1977). Intentional manipulation in the rewardingness of the environment is central to the community reinforcement approach (Hunt and Azrin 1973; Azrin 1976; Sisson and Azrin 1989), while the relevance of the patient's cultivation of substitute activities to processes of long-term recovery has been described by Vaillant (1983) and Edwards *et al.* (1992). The clinician is likely to be well aware that people do not stay away for long from drugs or alcohol if sobriety offers no more than a raw exposure to pain, or a vacuum of unfulfillment. Again, we do well to eschew the role of miracle worker—we cannot conjure up for everyone a happy marriage, a rewarding job, and an enriched leisure life, or the sun always shining, and we should not be edged into conniving with the notion that sobriety is only possible on those terms. Nonetheless, and as shown in Harald Klingemann's review of these issues (Chapter 8), persuasive evidence exists that qualities in the external environment can bear importantly on outcome. That must either provoke a sense of therapeutic pessimism or force us to ask questions as to how we are to enable our patients more effectively to engage with, and master, those externals. The message from the clinical frontline must, therefore, be that therapies which become abstract and too technical, and which forget that sobriety may be found through breeding budgerigars, taking up lessons in the Russian language, or teaching children to play football, have passed by an important aspect of what makes motivation. Closely allied to the notion of substitute activity is that of moving towards the ability to engage in, and taste rewards from behaviour which gives to others (Vaillant 1983). The exercise of altruism can be part of healing.

3. *Motivation and the therapeutic benefits which may derive from encouragement.* The significance of the therapeutic relationship has been extensively discussed in the generality of psychotherapy research (Truax and Carkhuff 1967; Frank 1973; Shapiro and Shapiro 1987; Lafferty *et al.* 1989), but to date this topic has received only scant attention in the specialist field of alcohol and drug research (Najavits and Weiss 1994): it is not, for instance, a theme which has been taken up at any length, in earlier chapters of the present book. Is the implicit message which is thus being given by researchers to practitioners in

the alcohol or drug clinics, that the practice of cognitive and behavioural techniques might equally well be carried out by a computer as by a human being?

The clinician would, of course, be expected to answer that query in the negative, if only out of desire to hold a job and not be rendered redundant by the machine. But if defensiveness is discounted, a number of important questions remain which should be directed back to the research community. The clinician would, for instance, probably argue that people who present with a severe drug or alcohol problem are often at that point rather specially discouraged and despairing, with their bad feelings about themselves a barrier to recovery. The experienced practitioner will then be likely further to suggest that in such circumstances clumsy therapeutics are marked by a wading in with a facile and cheery message which will carry no conviction, and which will rob the therapist of credibility. There are skills in knowing how to give encouragement without being in the process cloying (Edwards 1982). Giving hope is though, the clinician will argue, an essential part of the therapeutic business even if that aspect of motivation is not at present to be found dressed in the technical habiliments.

That awareness of the potential significance of the therapeutic relationship as a lever to recovery is not just a latter-day discovery, is shown by the following further quotation from Trotter's 'Essay on Drunkenness':

When the physician has once gained the full confidence of his patient, he will find little difficulty in beginning his plan of cure ... Particular opportunities are therefore to be taken, to hold up a mirror as it were, that he may see the deformity of his conduct, and represent the incurable maladies which flow from perseverance in a course of intemperance. There are times when a picture of this kind will make a strong impression on the mind; but at the conclusion of every visit, something consolatory must be left for amusement, and as food for his reflection. (Trotter 1804)

Motivational interviewing (Miller and Rollnick 1991), Trotter seems to be telling us, is not separable from the therapist–patient relationship, and the giving of hope is not something we should too readily leave to the computer.

HOW DO WE CONCEIVE OF, MEASURE, AND FACE UP TO CHANGE FOR THE WORSE?

In Chapter 6, Mary Alison Durand discusses the concept of 'Progressive disease', largely in relation to the image of 'alcoholism'. She suggests that:

While labels are obviously important, the danger is that in considering alcoholism as a progressive disease, we may become so preoccupied with the debate surrounding the usefulness or otherwise of the term 'disease', that we ignore the adjective 'progressive'.

It could be argued that although much effort has been directed at the measurement of the positive and beneficent outcomes which we hope to see unfold as consequences of treatment, research has in general shied away from the conceptual and measurement issues attaching to the negative and malign progress of deterioration. What is, as it were, the factor structure of change for the worse? This question is raised by John Strang (Chapter 12), when he discusses dimensions of harm. Jellinek's 'phases of alcoholism' (Jellinek 1952), represented an early attempt to map the progress of deterioration. It would though be too simple to assume that getting worse is to be understood simply as the obverse of getting better, and certain types of worsening (contraction of HIV infection, for instance), are a one-way track.

A categorical approach to this complex question is latent in the common phrasings 'early problem drinker', 'problem drinker', 'alcoholic', and 'chronic alcoholic'. An approach which segments continuous, multidimensional processes of change (Edwards 1984, 1989) into stages, phases, or other types of discontinuity, is though in this arena likely to be unhelpful—exactly the same point is made by Strang when discussing dimensions of improvement. Processes of change cannot be made into categories. Worsening, like getting better, is undoubtedly a dimensional and multidimensional process, rather than something which can be segmented into stages. Let us outline some of the types of change which may at times contribute to malign progression: they are types of process which need to be more fully understood both singly and in terms of their interaction, if we are better to comprehend deterioration. As Colin Taylor reminds us (Chapter 2), deterioration is sadly a large part of the play.

1. *Progress in degree of dependence*. We, at present, know hardly anything about progression in the degree of dependence in relation to any drug. We do not know whether dependence as measured, say, by the SADQ (Stockwell *et al.* 1979) or SODQ (Sutherland *et al.* 1986), predictably intensifies over time if the individual continues to drink or take drugs. Is worsening in dependence generally a straight line, exponential, asymptotic, or greatly variable by person, circumstance, or drug? Is regression likely to be intercut with progression, or

do morning shakes, once established, never go away and inevitably get worse? It is inconceivable that deterioration in this or any other regard will be found to be a matter of certainties. The need is empirically to establish the degrees of risk and likelihood.

2. *What progression occurs in the experience of depression?* Cross-sectional studies reveal that patients with drinking problems frequently report depressive symptoms (Schuckit *et al*. 1994). Perhaps about 40 per cent of such patients will, while drinking, manifest depression of such severity and continuance as to merit a diagnosis of depressive illness, although these symptoms will usually clear after a few weeks of abstinence (Brown and Schuckit 1988). What we do not know is whether the frequency or severity of depressive experience with drinking intensifies over time, with implications for social functioning, risk of suicide, or help seeking and recovery. Intensification over time in the affective element of withdrawal might be related to worsening in depression (Drummond 1990), and perhaps also to emergence of phobic symptoms (Stockwell *et al*. 1984). Similar time-based questions in relation to depression and the use of opiates and cocaine are equally unexplored.

3. *The significance of progressive brain damage.* Although the possibility of substance-related brain damage has been raised in relation to other drugs (Spencer and Boren 1990), by far the most clinically significant questions pertain here to alcohol (Oscar-Berman 1990). There are considerable data on the incidence of CAT scan abnormalities among patients with drinking problems, and an incidence as high as 40 per cent has been reported (Ron 1993). We know also that scan abnormalities can regress with abstinence, and progress with further drinking (Mann *et al*. 1993). What is less well charted is the likely speed of progression in brain damage with continued drinking, the variability in such progression between patients, with age, according to existing level of brain damage, and with intensity of drinking. We also know little about the implications of brain damage and associated impairment for impulse control, for further worsening in drinking behaviour, or for responsiveness to treatment (Gregson and Taylor 1977; Guthrie and Elliott 1980; Wilkinson and Sanchez-Craig 1981; Shaw and Spence 1985).

4. *Progressive deterioration in the social dimensions.* Deterioration may not only occur in the psychological and physical domains, but in relation to such issues as the individual's employability, loss of friends, or the intensity of involvement with a drinking or drug-taking

sub-culture. The most obvious externals of social deterioration are marked by, say, homelessness, divorce, or the prison sentence, but there are more subtle aspects in the social domain which need to be tracked, relating to the exclusion from normal society, social amplification of problems, and resultant difficulty in finding a way back to normality.

The sub-headings which have been given to the discussion above indicate only a few of many further possible types of happening or process which may on occasion contribute to things getting worse. The central point which we are seeking to make is that although the question of why people get better is a fruitful research topic (Edwards *et al.* 1988; Schuckit *et al.* 1986, 1993), the less attractive but clinically relevant questions relating to how and why people get worse, how we are to recognize worsening, and how deterioration is to be interdicted, are also very important. Sadly, the clinical frontline all too often sees people getting worse and even patients who are seemingly hell-bent on self-destruction. There are many studies which examine prognostic indicators for improvement, but few so far which dare approach the worrying, and highly important converse question. We need to know why drinkers kill themselves, why smokers smoke themselves to death, why injecting drug users continue to engage in unsafe sex or risky injecting practices, rather than dismissing these sad facts as just the dark side of 'good outcome'. Stephen Sutton's discussion of relapse in cigarette smokers (Chapter 7), speaks broadly to understanding of one important aspect of this question. Reginald Smart's discussion of 'escalation to dependence' in Chapter 5 deals with understanding of the early phase in the process of getting worse.

So much for a brief exploration of three themes relating to the building of bridges between research and clinical concerns in the substance problems world. There are many issues raised by earlier chapters of this book and which potentially bear on the application of science to real world problems, on which we have not even touched—the significance of biological understanding for future therapeutic developments for instance (Chapter 3), the economic dimensions (Chapter 9), the highly important question of how we are better to understand the population dissemination of habits (Chapter 10), and the all encompassing question of the relationship between science and policy (Chapter 11).

Taken together all these chapters amply and richly explore the change theme. Perhaps one ends up, in particular, persuaded that if the habiliments of science are not to become the emperor's new clothes, science had better listen rather closely to what the clinical world has inchoately to tell about change. And, equally, if the clinical world is to turn around, it had better listen to what science has to say about processes of change.

REFERENCES

Azrin, N. H. (1976). Improvements in the community reinforcement approach to Alcoholism. *Behaviour Research and Therapy*, **14**, 339–48.

Bien, T. H., Miller, W. R., and Tonigan, J. S. (1993). Brief interventions for alcohol problems: a review. *Addiction*, **88**, 315–36.

Birke, S. A., Edelmann, R. J., and Davis, P. E. (1990). An analysis of the abstinence violation effect in a sample of illicit drug users. *British Journal of Addiction*, **85**, 1299–307.

Brown, S. A. and Schuckit, M. A. (1988). Changes in depression among abstinent alcoholism. *Journal of Studies on Alcohol*, **49**, 412–17.

Drummond, D. C. (1990). The relationship between alcohol dependence and alcohol-related problems in a clinic population. *British Journal of Addiction*, **85**, 357–66.

Edwards, G. (1982). *The treatment of drinking problems: a guide for the helping professions*. McGraw Hill, New York.

Edwards, G. (1984). Drinking in longitudinal perspective: career and natural history. *British Journal of Addiction*, **79**, 175–83.

Edwards, G. (1989). As the years go rolling by: drinking problems in the time dimension. *British Journal of Psychiatry*, **154**, 18–26.

Edwards, G., Brown, D., Oppenheimer, E., Sheehan, M., Taylor, C., and Duckitt, A. (1988). Long-term outcome for patients with drinking problems: the search for predictors. *British Journal of Addiction*, **83**, 917–27.

Edwards, G., Oppenheimer, E., and Taylor, C. (1992). Hearing the noise in the system. Exploration of textual analysis as a method for studying change in drinking behaviour. *British Journal of Addiction*, **87**, 73–81.

Frank, J. D. (1973). *Persuasion and healing: a comparative study of psychiatry*, (Revised edition). Johns Hopkins University Press, Baltimore, MD.

Freeman, H. L. and Kendrick, D. C. (1960). A case of cat phobia. *British Medical Journal*, **2**, 497–502.

Gray, J. A. C. (1987). Interactions between drugs and behaviour therapy. In *Theoretical foundations in behaviour therapy* (ed. H. J. Eysenck and I. Martin), pp. 437–47. Plenum, New York.

Gregson, R. A. M. and Taylor, G. M. (1977). Prediction of relapse in male alcoholics. *Journal of Studies on Alcohol*, **38**, 1749–60.

Guthrie, A. and Elliott, W. A. (1980). The nature and reversibility of cerebral impairment in alcoholism: treatment implications. *Journal of Studies on Alcohol*, **41**, 147–55.

Hunt G. M. and Azrin, N. H. (1973). A community reinforcement approach to alcoholism. *Behaviour Research and Therapy*, **2**, 91–104.

Jarvis M. J. and Russell, M. A. H. (1989). Treatment for cigarette smoking. *International Review of Psychiatry*, **1**, 139–47.

Jellinek, E. M. (1952). Phases of alcoholism. *Quarterly Journal of Studies on Alcohol*, **13**, 673–84.

Klingemann, H. K-H. (1991). The motivation for change from problem alcohol and heroin use. *British Journal of Addiction*, **86**, 727–44.

Lafferty, P., Beuther, L., and Crago, M. (1989). Differences between more and less effective psychotherapists: a study of select therapist variables. *Journal of Consulting and Clinical Psychology*, **57**, 76–80.

Ludwig, A. M. (1985). Cognitive processes associated with 'spontaneous' recovery from alcoholism. *Journal of Studies on Alcohol*, **46**, 53–8.

Mann, K., Mundle, G., Langle, G., and Petersen, D. (1993). The reversibility of alcoholic brain damage is not due to rehydration: a CT study. *Addiction*, **88**, 649–54.

Marlatt, G. A. and Gordon, J. R. (ed.) (1985). *Relapse prevention: maintenance strategies in the treatment of addictive behaviour*. Guildford, New York.

Miller, W. R. (1989). Raiding the lost ark: do we need new models to study behavior change in spiritual contexts. *Spiritual and Religious Issues in Behavior Change*, **4**, 6–15.

Miller, W. R. and Hester, R. K. (1986). The effectiveness of alcoholism treatment: what research reveals. In *Treating addictive behaviors: processes of change* (ed. W. R. Miller and N. Heather), pp. 121–74. Plenum, New York.

Miller, W. R. and Rollnick, S. (1991). *Motivational interviewing: preparing people to change addictive behavior*. Guildford, New York.

Najavits, L. M. and Weiss, R. D. (1994). Variations in therapist effectiveness in the treatment of patients with substance use disorders: an empirical review. *Addiction*, **89**. (In press.)

O'Malley, S. S., Jaffe, A. J., Chang, G., Schollenfeld, R. S., Meyer, R. E., and Rounsaville, B. (1992). Naltrexone and coping skills therapy for alcohol dependence. A controlled study. *Archives of General Psychiatry*, **49**, 881–7.

Orford, J. (1977). Alcoholism: what psychology has to offer. In *Alcoholism, new knowledge and new responses* (ed. G. Edwards and M. Grant), pp. 88–9. Croom Helm, London.

Oscar-Berman, M. (1990). Learning and memory deficits in detoxified alcoholics, In *Residual effects of abused drugs in behavior* (ed. J. W. Spencer and J. J. Baren), pp. 136–55. US Department of Health and Human Services, Rockville, MD.

Prochaska, J. O. and Di Clemente, C. C. (1983). Stages and processes of self-change of smoking: toward an integrated model of change. *Journal of Consulting Clinical Psychology*, **51**, 390–5.

Rachman, S. and Hodgson, R. (1980). *Obsessions and compulsions*. Prentice Hall, Englewood Cliffs, NJ.

Richardson, B. W. (1883). *Diseases of modern life*. Fowler and Wells, New York.

Ron, M. A. (1983). The alcoholic brain: CT scan and psychological findings. *Psychological Medicine Supplement*, **3**, 1–32.

Saunders, J. B. (1989). The efficacy of treatment for drinking problems. *International Review of Psychiatry*, **1**, 121–38.

Saunders, B. and Wilkinson, C. (1990). Motivation and addiction behaviour. A psychological perspective. *Drug and Alcohol Review*, **9**, 133–43.

Schuckit, M. A., Schwell, M. G., and Gold, E. (1986). Prediction of outcome in inpatient alcoholics. *Quarterly Journal of Studies on Alcohol*, **47**, 151–5.

Schuckit, M. A., Smith, T. M., and Irwin, M. (1993). Subjective prediction of outcome among alcoholics. *Addiction*, **88**, 1361–7.

Schuckit, M. A., Irwin, M., and Smith, T. C. (1994). One-year incidence rate of major depression and other psychiatric disorders in 239 alcoholic men. *Addiction*, **89**, 441–6.

Shapiro, D. and Shapiro, D. A. (1987). Change processes in psychotherapy. *British Journal of Addiction*, **82**, 431–44.

Shaw, G. K. and Spence, (1985). Psychological impairment in alcoholics. *Alcohol and Alcoholism*, **20**, 243–9.

Sisson R. W. and Azrin, N. H. (1989). The community reinforcement approach. In *Handbook of alcoholism treatment approaches*, (ed. R. K. Hester and W. R. Miller), pp. 242–58. Pergamon, New York.

Sobell, L. C., Sobell, M. B., Toneatto, T., and Leo, G. I. (1993). What triggers the resolution of alcohol problems without treatment? *Alcoholism: Clinical and Experimental Research*, **17**, 217–24.

Spencer, J. W. and Boren, J. (ed.) (1990). *Residual effects of abused drugs on behavior. NIDA research monograph 101*. US Department of Health and Human Services, Rockville, MD.

Stitzer, M. L., Bigelow, G. E., and McCaul, M. E. (1983). Behavioral approaches to drug abuse. In Progress in behavioral modification, Vol. 14, (ed, M, Hersen, R. M. Eisler, and P. M. Miller), pp. 49–124. Academic Press, New York.

Stockwell, T., Hodgson, R., Edwards, G., Taylor, C., and Rankin, H. (1979). The development of a questionnaire to measure the severity of alcohol dependence. *British Journal of Addiction*, **74**, 79–87.

Stockwell, T., Smail, P., Hodgson, R., and Canter, S. (1984). Alcohol dependence and phobic states II. A retrospective study. *British Journal of Psychiatry*, **144**, 58–63.

Sutherland, G., Edwards, G., Taylor, C., Phillips, G., Gossop, M., and Brady, R. (1986). The measurement of opiate dependence. *British Journal of Addiction*, **81**, 534–48.

Trotter, T. (1804). *An essay, medical, philosophical and chemical, on drunkenness and its effects on the human body*. T. N. Longman and O. Rees, London.

Truax, C. B. and Carkhuff, R. R. (1967). *Toward effective counselling and psychotherapy*. Aldine, Chicago.

Tuchfeld, B. S. (1981). Spontaneous remission in alcoholics: empirical observations and theoretical implications. *Quarterly Journal of Studies on Alcohol*, **42**, 626–41.

Vaillant, G. E. (1983). *The natural history of alcoholism*. Harvard University Press, Cambridge, MA.

Wilkinson, D. A. and Sanchez-Craig, M. (1981). Relevance of brain dysfunction to treatment objectives: should alcohol-induced cognitive deficits influence the way we think about treatment? *Addictive Behavior*, **6**, 253–60.

Index